# Dr. Ruby Levine

# Empowered Women's

*A Complete Guide to Women's Health*

*This book was professionally typeset on Reedsy*
*Find out more at reedsy.com*

# Contents

1.

2.

    1.

      2.

3.

    1.

      2.

4.

    1.

      2.

5.

    1.

      2.

6.

    1.

      2.

7.

    1.

      2.

8.

    1.

      2.

9.

1.

2.

# Foreword

**Introduction**

Women's health is crucial for everyone's wellbeing as well as the development of society as a whole. The importance of women's health may be seen in a number of ways:

Personal Well-Being: Women's entire well-being and quality of life are strongly impacted by their health. Women who are in excellent health may live active, happy lives, pursue their objectives, and have satisfying connections with their families and communities.

Reproductive Health: Menstrual health, family planning, pregnancy, and delivery are all included in the category of reproductive health for women. Women are better able to make decisions about their bodies, reproductive options, and sexual health when they have access to reproductive healthcare services.

Maternal and Child Health: The wellbeing of mothers and their offspring are intertwined. Healthy women are more likely to have healthy pregnancies and to provide their children loving attention. It is essential to address women's health requirements throughout pregnancy and after delivery in order to lower maternal and newborn mortality rates and advance child development.

Women's health is a critical component of gender equality, which is a basic principle. To remove the hurdles and discrepancies that limit women's prospects and well-being, it is crucial to ensure that they have equitable access to healthcare services, information, and resources.

Economic Empowerment: Women who are in good health may work full-time and contribute to economic progress. When women have access to high-quality healthcare, their productivity rises, their absenteeism decreases, and their entire economic situation for themselves and their family improves.

Promoting preventative care and early disease diagnosis is a crucial part of placing women's health as a top priority. Regular exams, immunizations, and health checks can identify any problems early, enabling prompt treatment and better outcomes.

Women's health includes both their mental and emotional well-being in addition to their physical health. For women's general health and resilience, it is crucial to address mental health concerns, encourage self-care behaviors, and lessen stigma associated with asking for help.

Longevity and Aging: Healthy aging depends on women's health throughout the course of their lives. Menopause, osteoporosis, and cardiovascular health are just a few examples of age-related health issues that need to be addressed if you want to live independently and with a greater quality of life as you age.

Policy and Advocacy: By concentrating on women's health, lobbying initiatives and policy alterations that improve healthcare systems, expand access to services, and take care of gender-specific health requirements are encouraged. It emphasizes the value of research, money, and laws that put women's health first.

Societies may promote a more fair and inclusive environment where women can flourish, contribute, and reach their full potential by giving women's health first priority. Not only is it the moral thing to do to invest in women's health, but it also has major social, economic, and public health advantages.

# 1

# Knowledge of the Female Body

This chapter gives a thorough description of the female body's structure, physiology, and distinctive features. Women must have a thorough understanding of the female anatomy in order to make wise choices regarding their health and well-being.

1.The female reproductive system is examined in detail in this section, including its organs and processes. Explaining how the ovaries, Fallopian tubes, uterus, cervix, and vagina function in monthly cycles, ovulation, fertilization, and pregnancy, it covers a variety of issues.

2. Hormonal Changes: In this section, we'll talk about the hormonal changes a woman experiences during her life, such as puberty, menstruation, and menopause. It discusses the function of hormones like progesterone and estrogen and how their variations affect both physical and mental health.

3. Menstruation and Menstrual Health: In this part, menstruation and menstrual health are the main topics. The menstrual cycle, typical menstrual problems, and management strategies are all covered.

period cleanliness, period products, typical monthly symptoms, and when to seek medical help are all covered.

4. Breast Health: Knowing the female body requires an awareness of breast health. The anatomy of the breasts, breast self-examinations, mammography, and interpreting breast changes are all covered in this section. The significance of early detection and routine breast health examinations is emphasized.

5. Sexual and Reproductive Health: In this part, we look at sexual and reproductive health. We discuss things like sexual anatomy, sexual pleasure, contraception, STIs, and typical reproductive health issues. It offers advice on healthy and safe sexual behavior and places a strong emphasis on the value of communication and consent.

6. Osteoporosis and Bone Health: Bone health is important for women, especially as they age. The significance of calcium, vitamin D, and exercise for keeping strong bones is covered in this section. Additionally included are osteoporosis' risk factors, therapeutic options, and preventative measures.

7. Urinary Health: Women frequently have urinary health issues, including urinary tract infections (UTIs) and pelvic floor health. This section offers guidance on preserving urinary health, identifying symptoms, obtaining treatment, and taking preventative actions.

8. Body Image and Self-Esteem: This section looks at how cultural expectations affect people's perceptions of their bodies and their self-worth. It covers methods for fostering self-esteem, creating a positive body image, and creating a good relationship with one's body.

9. Genetics and Women's Health: Genetic factors can affect the problems and hazards associated with women's health. The influence of genetics on reproductive and medical decisions, as well as genetic testing and hereditary diseases, is discussed in this section.

In order to preserve good health and make wise decisions, it is crucial to understand the female body, which is stressed in this chapter's conclusion. It lays the groundwork for the later chapters, which will dig more deeply into particular facets of women's health and well-being.

**The reproductive system in women**

The female reproductive system is a unique and sophisticated mechanism that produces eggs (ova), promotes fertilization, sustains pregnancy, and facilitates childbirth. For women's health and reproductive well-being, it is crucial to understand the female reproductive system. Let's examine the essential elements and capabilities of the female reproductive system:

1. Ovaries: On either side of the uterus are two almond-shaped organs known as the ovaries. They go through a procedure called

ovulation to generate and release eggs (ova). Additionally, progesterone and estrogen, which control the menstrual cycle and aid in the maturation of secondary sexual traits, are produced by the ovaries.

2. Fallopian Tubes: The Fallopian tubes connect the ovaries to the uterus and are also referred to as uterine tubes or oviducts. The eggs can go through these tubes from the ovaries to the uterus. Usually, the union of a sperm and an egg takes place inside the Fallopian tubes.

3. Uterus: A fertilized egg implants in the uterus, sometimes referred to as the womb, where it grows into a fetus throughout pregnancy. The uterus is made up of three layers: the perimetrium, the myometrium, which is the middle layer of muscle, and the endometrium, which is the innermost layer of lining.

4. Cervix: The lower end of the uterus, which links to the vagina, is known as the cervix. It acts as a passageway between the body's inside and exterior. The cervix widens during delivery to provide room for the baby to pass through.

5. Vagina: The muscular channel that joins the cervix to the external genitalia is known as the vagina. It allows sexual activity, works as the birth canal during delivery, and acts as a conduit for menstrual blood flow.

6. Vulva: The term "vulva" refers to the exterior female genitalia, which includes the clitoris, labia majora, and labia minora. It offers defense and contains delicate nerve endings linked to sex pleasure.

7. Menstrual Cycle: A hormonal and physiological process, the menstrual cycle gets the body ready for a future pregnancy. Generally speaking, it lasts for around 28 days, however it might vary from person to person. The uterine lining thickens throughout the menstrual cycle in order to prepare for the implantation of a fertilized egg. In the absence of fertilization, the lining sheds, causing monthly bleeding.

8. Hormonal Control: Hormones have a complex role in controlling the female reproductive system. Estrogen and progesterone, which are largely generated by the ovaries, are the major hormones at play. These hormones are essential for maintaining reproductive health, controlling secondary sexual characteristics, and regulating the menstrual cycle.

For women to make educated decisions about contraception, family planning, reproductive health, and fertility, they must have a thorough understanding of the female reproductive system. Regular examinations and screenings, such mammograms and Pap tests, can help identify possible problems and guarantee early action, enhancing general reproductive well-being.

# Hormonal Changes and the Menstrual Cycle

In women of reproductive age, the menstrual cycle is a normal process that involves a number of hormonal and physiological changes in anticipation of a prospective pregnancy. Although there are many variances, the average duration is about 28 days. Women may manage their reproductive health, track their fertility, and comprehend the changes taking place in their bodies by understanding the menstrual cycle and the hormonal changes that go along with each phase. Let's examine the important menstrual cycle phases and the hormonal changes linked to each stage:

1. Menstruation (Days 1–5): Menstruation, or endometrial shedding when there is no pregnancy, marks the start of the monthly cycle. The two main female reproductive hormones, progesterone and estrogen, are at their lowest levels at this time. Prostaglandins are released when hormone levels fall, which causes the uterus to contract and remove the lining, causing monthly bleeding.

2. Follicular Phase (Days 1–14): The follicular phase starts after menstruation. Follicle-stimulating hormone (FSH), which is released by the pituitary gland during this phase, encourages the development of many follicles in the ovaries. Undeveloped eggs are found inside each follicle. The follicles generate estrogen as they develop, in order to prepare the endometrium for prospective implantation of a fertilized egg. The dominant follicle often advances while the others regress.

3. Ovulation (about Day 14): Ovulation is the release of an egg that has reached maturity from the ovary. A spike in luteinizing hormone

(LH), which the pituitary gland also secretes, causes it to occur. The dominant follicle bursts as a result of the LH surge, delivering the egg into the Fallopian tube. Ovulation, which occurs around day 14 of a 28-day cycle, is the most fertile period of the menstrual cycle. The cervical mucus becomes thinner and more elastic as estrogen levels rise, which promotes sperm survival and motility.

4. Luteal Phase (Days 15–28): The ovary's burst follicle develops into a transient gland known as the corpus luteum following ovulation. Progesterone, which is produced by the corpus luteum, gets the uterus ready for possible implantation of a fertilized egg. To make the endometrium thicker and better suited for embryo implantation, progesterone is used. The corpus luteum continues to generate progesterone to support early pregnancy if fertilization does place. In the absence of fertilization, the corpus luteum degenerates, which lowers hormone levels.

5. Premenstrual Phase (Days 25–28): If pregnancy does not occur, hormone levels, notably progesterone, start to fall in the days before menstruation. Some women may experience a variety of premenstrual symptoms due to this drop in hormone levels, including mood swings, bloating, breast soreness, and fatigue.

A complex interaction of hormones, including estrogen, progesterone, FSH, and LH, controls the menstrual cycle. These hormones control how the follicles grow and mature, how the eggs are released, and how the uterus gets ready for a future pregnancy. Understanding the menstrual cycle and the hormonal changes it causes can help women spot anomalies, monitor their fertility, and, if necessary, seek the right medical guidance.

**Teenage Health and Puberty**

A crucial developmental stage that separates infancy from maturity is puberty. It is a time when both boys and girls experience significant physical, emotional, and psychological changes as a result of hormonal changes. To successfully traverse this transitional time, young people, their parents, and caregivers must have a solid understanding of puberty and adolescent health. Let's go more into puberty and teenage health:

1. Puberty: For girls, puberty normally starts between the ages of 8 and 14 and for boys, between the ages of 9 and 16. Hormones, typically estrogen in females and testosterone in males, are released to start it. Puberty brings about a number of significant changes, such as:

Physical changes include growth spurts, the commencement of menstruation in girls, changes in body form, and the development of secondary sexual traits in both boys and girls, such as the development of breasts in girls and facial hair in boys.

- Development of the reproductive system: The reproductive organs mature and the capacity to conceive and procreate grows.

- Emotional and Psychological Changes: Adolescents could go through mood swings, acquire a stronger sense of who they are, become more self-aware, or develop a sexual desire.

2. Menstruation and Menstrual Health: For girls, menstruation frequently begins during adolescence. The need of teaching young girls about menstruation, its function, and how to handle it hygienically cannot be overstated. Promoting girls' menstrual health include talking about menstrual hygiene products, addressing typical worries and pain, and promoting open discussions about periods.

3. Emotional and Mental Health: Adolescence may be an emotionally and psychologically taxing time. Stress, anxiety, and mood disorders can be exacerbated by hormonal fluctuations, peer pressure, academic requirements, and body image problems. Supporting teenage emotional well-being requires fostering open communication, offering emotional support, and developing good coping methods.

4. Comprehensive Sexual and Reproductive Health Education: Adolescence is an ideal period to deliver sexual and reproductive health information. It is important to talk about issues like puberty, physical changes, sexual health, contraception, STIs, consent, and healthy relationships. Adolescents can experience fewer STIs and fewer unwanted pregnancies by learning about responsible sexual conduct and safe procedures.

5. Nutrition and Exercise: Adolescent health depends on a balanced diet and frequent exercise. Physical exercise encourages healthy bones, muscles, and overall wellbeing, while proper diet supports healthy growth and development. Promoting a nutritious diet and an active lifestyle lowers the chance of developing chronic illnesses, prevents obesity, and fosters a good self-image.

6. Substance Abuse and dangerous habits: Adolescents may experience peer pressure and experiment with dangerous habits including smoking, drinking alcohol, or using drugs. Adolescents can be protected against substance misuse and its harmful effects by being informed about the hazards involved, encouraging healthy coping mechanisms, and creating a supportive environment.

7. Preventive healthcare: It's crucial for adolescents to have routine medical exams, vaccines, and screenings. Health care providers can keep an eye on development and growth and respond quickly to any problems. Vaccinations offer defense against several malignancies and STIs, including the HPV vaccination for boys and girls. Encouragement of routine medical visits fosters the development of a lifetime preventive healthcare habit.

8. Consent and Healthy Relationships: It's important to teach teenagers about consent, setting boundaries, and promoting healthy relationships. Promotes their safety and wellbeing by teaching kids about respect, communication, and spotting abusive or unhealthy relationships.

Promoting adolescent health and wellbeing requires supportive settings, open communication, and availability of correct information. Helping adolescents manage the difficulties and changes of puberty requires empowering them with knowledge, offering emotional support, and building a secure and inclusive atmosphere.

Promoting adolescent health and wellbeing requires supportive settings, open communication, and availability of correct information. Helping adolescents manage the difficulties and changes of puberty requires empowering them with knowledge, offering emotional support, and building a secure and inclusive atmosphere.

*Obstetrics and childbirth*

Birthing a child and becoming pregnant are life-changing events that result in the production of new life. The expecting woman experiences several physical, mental, and hormonal changes throughout this amazing journey. For women and their partners to have a successful and satisfying pregnancy, prenatal care, labor, and postpartum recovery, knowledge is essential. Let's go further into pregnancy and delivery:

1. Pregnancy: A fertilized egg attaches itself in the uterus where it grows into an embryo and then a fetus, signaling the start of pregnancy. Pregnancy lasts an average of 40 weeks, broken up into three trimesters:

- First Trimester (Weeks 1–12): The body goes through a lot of changes during this time as the embryo grows into a fetus. Fatigue, morning sickness, breast soreness, and frequent urination are typical early pregnancy symptoms. To keep track of the mother's and the unborn child's health, early prenatal care is crucial.

The second trimester, which lasts from weeks 13 to 27, is sometimes referred to as the "honeymoon phase" of pregnancy. The majority of women report lessening of the early pregnancy symptoms and an increase in energy. The fetus is still developing, and The mother starts to feel fetal movements as the fetus develops more. To track the development of the unborn child and identify any possible issues, prenatal screenings and ultrasounds may be carried out.

- Third Trimester (Weeks 28–40+): The fetus develops and gains weight quickly throughout the third trimester. Shortness of breath, backaches, edema, and the mother's enlarged uterus may all cause pain. More regular prenatal checkups are necessary to monitor the baby's position, evaluate the mother's health, and get ready for delivery.

2. Prenatal Care: To protect the health and wellbeing of both the mother and the unborn child, prenatal care entails frequent medical

checkups and assistance during pregnancy. Physical inspections, weight and blood pressure checks, fetal monitoring, and other procedures are frequently performed during prenatal appointments, screening exams, too. Nutritional counseling, prenatal education, and birth preference conversations are all included in prenatal care.

3. Childbirth: The process of bringing a baby out of the mother's womb and into the world is referred to as childbirth. Depending on the mother's health, the position of the baby, and other variables, it may happen via a variety of methods, such as vaginal birth or cesarean section (C-section). Create a birth plan with the help of your healthcare providers if you want to express your preferences for things like labor support, pain relief, and the environment during labor and delivery.

- Vaginal Birth: During a vaginal birth, the woman undergoes labor, which consists of three phases - the dilatation and effacement of the cervix, the pushing stage, and the delivery of the placenta following the baby's birth, Breathing exercises, relaxation techniques, and medicine are all possible pain treatment strategies.

- Cesarean section (C-section): A C-section is a surgical operation in which the mother's abdomen and uterus are cut, allowing the baby to be delivered. Usually, it is advised when a vaginal birth might endanger the woman or the unborn child.

4. Postpartum Recovery: The time following childbirth, known as the postpartum phase, requires the mother to make both physical and

mental adaptations as her body recovers from pregnancy and childbirth and adjusts to its new normal. Managing postpartum discomfort, aiding breastfeeding, emotional health, and developing a routine for baby care are all possible aspects of postpartum recovery. During this time of change, it is critical for women to have support from medical professionals, family, and friends.

Every woman's experience with pregnancy and delivery is distinct, and these experiences are unique. obtaining prenatal care, learning about your alternatives,

## Aging and Menopause

The menopause, a biologically normal process, signals the end of a woman's fertile years. Menstrual cycles stop, and the synthesis of reproductive hormones, especially estrogen and progesterone, decreases. Menopause normally happens between the ages of 45 and 55, however each person's timing may vary. Aging is a natural process that impacts both men and women, along with menopause. Let's delve more into menopause and aging:

1. Menopause: Perimenopause is a transitional stage that frequently precedes menopause. Perimenopause is characterized by hormonal fluctuations and the potential for irregular menstruation. Menopause symptoms might include the following:

Hot flashes: An abrupt sense of heat that is frequently accompanied by flushing and perspiration.

- Night sweats: Excessive perspiration while you sleep that may interfere with your sleep schedule.

- Vaginal dryness: Reduced lubrication and weakening of the tissues in the vaginal area, which causes pain during sexual activity.

- Mood swings, impatience, and changes in emotional well-being can all be attributed to hormonal fluctuations.

- Sleep disturbances: Hormone changes and night sweats can interfere with sleep cycles and cause insomnia.

- Modifications in sexual function: Libido and sexual arousal may change as a result of low estrogen levels.

- Urinary symptoms such as increased frequency, urgency, or incontinence may be experienced by certain women due to changes in their urinary system.

2. Health Considerations During Menopause: It is crucial for women to put their health and wellbeing first both during and after menopause. Among the most important factors are:

- Bone health: Lower estrogen levels can cause bone density to decline, raising the risk of osteoporosis. To preserve bone health, it's critical to concentrate on calcium-rich meals, vitamin D, and weight-bearing workouts. In such circumstances, doctors may advise hormone treatment and bone density tests to control bone health.

- Heart health: Women's risk of developing heart disease may rise after menopause. Cardiovascular health depends on leading a heart-healthy lifestyle, which includes regular exercise, a balanced diet, keeping a healthy weight, controlling cholesterol and blood pressure levels, and quitting smoking.

- Breast health: Routine mammography and breast self-exams are essential for spotting any alterations or anomalies in breast tissue. It is crucial to go over breast cancer screening recommendations with medical professionals.

- Mental and emotional health: Hormonal changes associated with menopause may have an effect on mood and emotional health. For general well-being, it is crucial to seek assistance, live a healthy lifestyle, and discuss any mental health issues with healthcare professionals.

3. Aging: Regardless of gender, aging is a normal process that affects everyone. Key characteristics of aging include:

- Physical changes: As people age, their physical characteristics may alter, including wrinkles, gray hair, and changes in the flexibility of their skin. Healthy aging may be promoted by leading a healthy lifestyle that includes a balanced diet, frequent exercise, and good skincare.

- Cognitive changes: As people age, some cognitive changes, such minor memory lapses, may take place. Social interaction, cognitively challenging hobbies, and leading a healthy lifestyle may all help with cognitive health.

- Chronic illness management: As people age, their chance of getting chronic conditions including heart disease, diabetes, and some malignancies rises. A healthy lifestyle, preventative screenings, and routine medical exams are crucial for controlling and lowering the risk of chronic illnesses.

- Emotional health: As we age, our emotions may vary and shift. The key to emotional well-being is creating a solid support network, taking part in activities that make you happy and fulfilled, and getting mental health care when you need it.

# 2

# Keeping up Physical

For general well-being and quality of life, maintaining physical health is essential. You will receive in-depth knowledge and useful advice in this chapter to help you focus and improve your physical health. You may improve your physical well-being by developing healthy habits, getting regular exercise, eating right, and putting preventative care first.

Section 1: Fitness and Exercise

1. The advantages of exercise

- Better cardiovascular health - Increased power, flexibility, and stamina

- Controlling one's weight - Reducing stress and enhancing mental health - Reducing the chance of developing chronic diseases

- An increase in vigor and general energy

2. Exercise styles: - Aerobic workouts for cardiovascular health, such as running, swimming, and cycling

- Strengthening workouts that increase bone density and muscular strength, such as weightlifting

- Flexibility activities to increase range of motion and avoid injuries, such as yoga and stretching

- Balance and coordination activities for stability and fall prevention, such as tai chi and balance training

3. Creating an Exercise Program:

- Based on your level of fitness and your tastes, set reasonable targets.

- Use a variety of workouts to focus on various muscle groups.

- Gradually increase time and intensity to prevent overexertion - Think about seeking advice from a fitness expert for specific recommendations

Section 2: Nutrition and Optimal Eating Patterns,

Diet that is balanced:

Include a range of fruits, vegetables, whole grains, lean meats, and healthy fats in your diet.

- Reduce your intake of processed meals, sugary snacks, and sugary beverages.

- Maintain your hydration by consuming enough water.

2. Portion Control: - Use smaller plates and bowls to regulate portion sizes - Practice mindful eating and pay attention to your body's hunger and fullness cues

- Pay attention to calorie-dense meals and keep portion amounts in check.

3. Nutritional Considerations: - Make sure you're getting enough of the nutrients you need, including vitamins, minerals, and antioxidants.

- Take into account any dietary demands or limits (e.g., allergies, intolerances, or medical issues).

If required, speak with a licensed dietician for individualized advice.

Section 3: Health Screenings and Preventive Care

1. Consistent Checkups:

- Make regular appointments with the doctor to check on your general health.

- Talk about the precautions and tests that are suitable for your age and gender.

2. Vaccinations: Maintain current immunization records to prevent infectious illnesses.

3. Early detection and screening:

- Adhere to advice for screening procedures such mammograms, Pap smears, colonoscopies, and cholesterol tests.

- If you have any unsettling symptoms or changes in your health, see a doctor right once.

Conclusion: You may maintain and enhance your physical health by prioritizing exercise, establishing a good diet, and taking preventative care. Remember to tailor these suggestions to your own need and seek the advice of medical specialists for specialized advice. Making physical fitness a priority will result in a healthier and more

**Women's Nutrition and Balanced Diet**

For women to support their general health, maintain energy levels, control weight, and lower the risk of chronic illnesses, proper nutrition and a balanced diet are crucial. Here are some important factors to keep in mind for women-only nutrition and a balanced diet:

1. Macro-nutrients: - carbs: Opt for complex carbs, which offer sustaining energy and crucial nutrients, such whole grains, legumes, fruits, and vegetables.

   - Protein: To promote muscle growth, repair, and general health, consume lean sources of protein such poultry, fish, eggs, beans, and tofu.

   - Fats: Choose healthy fats from foods like olive oil, nuts, seeds, and avocados. Limit the intake of processed snacks and fried meals that contain saturated and trans fats.

2. Micro-nutrients: - Iron: Women require more iron, particularly while menstruating and pregnant. Lean meats, beans, lentils, leafy greens, and fortified cereals are some examples of foods high in iron.

   - Calcium and vitamin D: For healthy bones and teeth, a diet rich in calcium and vitamin D is essential. Be sure to eat dairy products, plant-based milk with added vitamins, leafy greens, and fatty fish.

- Folate: Beneficial for female reproductive health, particularly during pregnancy. Include foods high in folate, such as leafy greens, citrus fruits, legumes, and cereals with added folate.

The omega-3 fatty acids Omega-3 fatty acids, which are included in walnuts and fatty fish (such as salmon and trout), promote heart health, cognitive function, and decrease inflammation.

3. Fiber: Consume fiber-rich foods including whole grains, fruits, vegetables, legumes, nuts, and seeds to aid digestion, control blood sugar levels, and keep a healthy weight.

4. Hydration: To keep hydrated and maintain general physiological functioning, drink enough of water throughout the day.

5. Adequate Caloric Intake: - Consume the right number of calories for your age, level of exercise, and general health objectives to meet your body's energy requirements. To receive individualized advice, speak with a qualified dietician.

6. Limit Added Sugars and Processed meals: - Reduce your intake of processed meals, sugary drinks, sweets, and other items rich in added sugar.

7. Meal planning and portion control: - Plan meals ahead of time to guarantee a range of nutrients and balanced meals.

- Use portion control to keep your weight in check and prevent overeating.

8. Factors to Take into Account During Different Life Stages: - Pregnancy and Lactation: Women who are pregnant or nursing have higher nutritional demands. For more detailed advice, speak with a qualified dietician or medical professional.

- Menopause: To maintain bone health and manage hormonal fluctuations, put an emphasis on calcium-rich diets, whole grains, lean proteins, and foods containing phytoestrogens (like soy).

Remember that each woman may have different dietary requirements depending on her age, degree of exercise, and underlying medical issues. A licensed dietitian or other healthcare professional can help you develop a customized nutrition plan that meets your unique requirements and objectives.

## Women's Fitness and Exercise

Fitness and exercise are essential for the general health and wellbeing of women. Regular exercise lowers the chance of developing chronic illnesses, improves cardiovascular health, elevates mood, and helps maintain a healthy weight. Several important factors for women's fitness and exercise are listed below:

1. Cardiovascular Exercise: - Take part in aerobic exercises including dance, jogging, cycling, swimming, or brisk walking.

- Aim for 75 minutes of severe aerobic activity or at least 150 minutes of moderate aerobic exercise each week.

- Engage in enjoyable activities to make it more enjoyable and sustainable.

2. Strength Training: Include workouts that will help you develop and maintain your muscular strength.

Use body weight workouts, free weights, weight machines, resistance bands, or other equipment.

- Include movements like squats, lunges, push-ups, and rows that focus on main muscular groups.

- Aim for strength training on at least two days each week.

3. Flexibility and Stretching: Incorporate stretching exercises to increase joint range of motion, flexibility, and to ward against ailments.

- Include static stretches for the major muscle groups, either as a post-workout regimen or as a stand-alone exercise.

- Take into account exercises that enhance flexibility, balance, and core strength, such as yoga or Pilates.

Include activities that work the core muscles (abdominals, lower back, and pelvic floor) in your workout routine.

- Examples of core workouts include planks, crunches, pelvic floor exercises (Kegels), and yoga positions like the boat posture.

- Posture, stability, and general body strength are all supported by a strong core.

5. Balance and Stability: Include activities that increase balance and stability, lowering the possibility of accidents and injuries.

- Incorporate yoga, tai chi, or particular balancing exercises like heel-to-toe walking or single-leg standing.

6. Pay Attention to Your Body's Cues: - Pay attention to your body's signals and alter your workouts or intensity as necessary.

- Take a break when you need to to avoid overexertion and injury.

7. Stay Active Throughout the Day: - Look for ways to stay active throughout the day, such as using the stairs, biking or walking short distances instead of driving, or inserting movement breaks into sedentary tasks.

8. Seek Professional Guidance: Speak with a fitness expert or personal trainer to create a customized workout program based on your objectives, degree of fitness, and any unique factors.

9. Pregnancy and Postpartum Considerations: - Talk with your healthcare provider throughout pregnancy to identify the best workouts and adaptations.

- Following childbirth, begin slowly getting back into shape as your healthcare professional advises, keeping in mind postpartum recovery and any particular instructions or limits.

If you've never exercised before, keep in mind that you should start slowly and build up your time and intensity over time. Make sure to find things you love and include regular exercise into your daily life. To prevent overworking yourself or being hurt, put safety first and pay attention to your body.

**Controlling one's weight and body image**

Important issues like body image and weight control may have a big influence on a woman's physical and mental health. The following are some ideas and tactics for preserving a healthy weight and encouraging a positive body image:

1. Prioritize Overall Health: - Prioritize overall health and well-being rather than only focusing on weight. Work toward living a balanced lifestyle that includes regular exercise, a healthy diet, enough sleep, stress management, and self-care.

Instead of aiming for an unattainable or unhealthy body size or form, set realistic and achievable objectives for your health and well-being.
   - Do not compare your own standards to those that are projected in the media or on social media.

3. Healthy Eating Habits: - Adopt an eating plan that is well-balanced and nutrient-dense and that contains a range of whole foods, including fruits, vegetables, lean meats, whole grains, and healthy fats.
   - By observing your hunger and fullness cues, eating gently, and appreciating the tastes of your meals, you may practice mindful eating.

4. Consistent Physical exercise: - Consistently engage in physical exercise that you find enjoyable and that fits with your skills and interests.

- Instead of concentrating exclusively on calorie burning, place an emphasis on developing strength, endurance, flexibility, and cardiovascular fitness.

5. Exercise self-compassion and body acceptance:

- Accept and value your body for its power, usefulness, and distinctive features.

- Refrain from speaking negatively about yourself or acting in body-shaming ways.

- To promote a good body image, practice self-compassion and affirmations.

6. Surround Yourself with Positive Influences: - Surround yourself with encouraging and upbeat people who encourage acceptance of one's physique and self-love.

- Reduce your exposure to media and social media that promote unrealistic beauty standards or messages about having a poor body image.

7. Seek Professional Support: If you're having issues with your body image, you might want to go to a therapist or counselor who focuses on these issues.

8. Avoid Fad Diets or Extreme Measures: - Focus on creating sustainable, long-term lifestyle changes that promote overall health

and well-being rather to using fad diets, extreme weight reduction techniques, or other practices that might harm your physical or mental health.

There is no one "ideal" body size or form because each body is different. Prioritizing self-care, body acceptance, and general wellness over aiming for society or unattainable norms is crucial. Positivity about one's body image and general wellbeing may be enhanced by concentrating on self-love and self-acceptance and developing a healthy connection with one's body.

*Preventing and Treating Common Health Problems*

Women might have common health problems at different phases of life. Following are some important health conditions, along with suggested preventative measures and therapeutic options:

First, breast health

- Prevention: Follow the advice of healthcare professionals and schedule routine clinical breast exams, mammograms, and breast self-examinations.

- Treatment: Medication, hormonal treatment, surgery, radiation, and chemotherapy are all possibilities for treating breast diseases.

2. Heart disease: - Prevention: Lead a heart-healthy lifestyle by eating a balanced diet, getting regular exercise, handling stress, quitting smoking, and keeping an eye on your cholesterol and blood pressure levels.

- Treatment: Depending on the severity of the problem, treatment may entail a change in lifestyle, medication, cardiac treatments, or surgery.

3. Osteoporosis: - Prevention: Eat a calcium-rich diet, do weight-bearing activities, make sure your vitamin D levels are appropriate, abstain from smoking and drinking too much alcohol, and think about getting your bone density checked.

- Options for treatment include hormone therapy, calcium and vitamin D supplements, drugs to increase bone density, and lifestyle changes.

4. Mental Health: - Prevention: Give self-care, stress management, consistent exercise, normal sleep patterns, and assistance from family members or mental health specialists a high priority.

- Treatment: Therapy, counseling, medication, lifestyle modifications, and support from mental health specialists may all be used to treat mental health disorders.

5. Reproductive health (including polycystic ovarian syndrome (PCOS), irregular menstruation, etc.):

- Prevention: Lead a healthy lifestyle, control your stress, keep a healthy weight, and consult a doctor if you have severe menstruation abnormalities or other PCOS-related symptoms.

- Treatment: To control symptoms and enhance reproductive health, treatment options may include hormone therapy, lifestyle changes, and medication.

6. Sexual and reproductive health (including use of contraception and STDs):

- Prevention: Engage in healthy sexual behavior, including the use of barrier techniques like condoms, routine STI testing, and STI vaccinations like HPV.

- Treatment: Depending on the individual infection, there are many STI treatment options, including medication, counseling, and lifestyle changes. There are several reliable ways of birth control, including hormonal, barrier, and intrauterine devices.

7. Cancer (such as uterine, ovarian, and cervical):

- Prevention: Be aware of family history, have regular screenings including Pap smears and HPV testing for cervical cancer, keep a healthy lifestyle, and consult a doctor if any symptoms are worrisome.

- Treatment: Depending on the kind and stage of the disease, treatment options for cancer can range from surgery to radiation therapy to chemotherapy to targeted therapy to immunotherapy.

It's vital to keep in mind that controlling and treating a variety of health concerns requires prevention, early discovery, and immediate medical intervention. It's critical to have regular check-ups, screenings, and open contact with medical professionals. Consult with healthcare specialists for individualized counsel and assistance based on your unique situation since each health condition may call for particular remedies.

**Cardiovascular disease and cardiovascular health**

For women, cardiovascular health is a crucial component of general wellbeing. One of the main causes of death for women is heart disease, which is a prevalent worry. It is essential to comprehend cardiovascular health and take preventive action. The following are important details about cardiovascular health and heart disease in women:

1. Risk elements
   - High blood pressure: If necessary, take medication and make lifestyle changes to maintain a healthy blood pressure level.
   - High cholesterol: Keep a close eye on your cholesterol levels and follow a heart-healthy diet that limits your intake of saturated and trans fats.
   - Smoking: Steer clear of smoking and passive smoking.
   - Obesity: Keep a healthy weight by eating a balanced diet and engaging in regular exercise.
   - Diabetes: Control diabetes by controlling blood sugar levels and collaborating with healthcare professionals.
   - Family history: Inform healthcare professionals about any history of heart disease in your family.

2. A heart-healthy lifestyle includes: - Eating a balanced diet that includes a range of fruits, vegetables, whole grains, lean meats, and

heart-healthy fats. Reduce your intake of processed meals, sweet snacks, and drinks.

- Regular exercise: Spend at least 150 minutes each week participating in aerobic activities such brisk walking, running, cycling, or swimming. Include workouts that build strength as well.

- Stress reduction: Use relaxation methods to reduce your stress levels, such as yoga, meditation, and deep breathing.

- Getting enough sleep: Aim for 7-8 hours of good sleep each night.

- Moderate alcohol usage or abstain from it completely.

- Schedule routine checkups with medical professionals for screenings, evaluations, and preventative treatment.

3. Recognize the following red flags: Be mindful of probable heart disease symptoms in women, which may be different from those frequently observed in males. These include discomfort or pain in the chest, shortness of breath, exhaustion, dizziness, nausea, pain in the jaw or back, and unusual perspiration. If you have any unsettling symptoms, speak with a medical professional.

4. Screening and diagnostic procedures: - Go through routine health examinations, such as blood pressure checks, cholesterol measurements, and diabetes tests.

- Additional tests like electrocardiograms (ECG), stress tests, echo-cardiograms, or coronary angiography could be advised by medical professionals depending on age and personal risk factors.

5. Treatment and Management: - Depending on the exact condition and severity, many treatments are available for heart disease. They might involve a change in lifestyle, medication, heart surgery (such as a bypass or valve repair), angioplasty, placing stents, or other cardiac treatments.

- To create a tailored treatment plan and implement it effectively, work together with healthcare professionals.

6. Education and Awareness: - Keep up to date on heart health, heart disease, and the special needs of female patients.

- To increase comprehension and enhance decision-making, take part in educational programs, look for trustworthy information sources, and have conversations with healthcare professionals.

Remember that sustaining cardiovascular health depends on early identification, preventative actions, and rapid medical intervention. Reducing the risk of heart disease and enhancing general cardiovascular well-being need regular contact with healthcare practitioners and active engagement in heart-healthy lifestyle choices.

**Osteoporosis and Bone Wellness**

Women need strong, healthy bones as they age, and osteoporosis is a prevalent disorder that compromises bone density and strength. Here are some important details concerning osteoporosis and bone health:

1. The significance of bone health: Bones aid in mobility, protect internal organs, and offer structural support.

- Adequate amounts of calcium, vitamin D, and other minerals are necessary for strong bones.

- Bone health maintenance is essential for avoiding fractures and osteoporosis.

2. Osteoporosis Risk Factors: - Age: Osteoporosis risk rises with age, especially after menopause.

- Gender: Women are more vulnerable than males, especially after the menopause when hormones fluctuate.

- Family history: The risk is increased if there is a history of osteoporosis in the family.

- Petite frame and low body weight: Women who have these characteristics are more vulnerable.

- Sedentary lifestyle: Bone loss might be exacerbated by a lack of weight-bearing activity.

- Smoking and binge drinking both have a detrimental effect on bone health.

3. Establishing and Preserving Healthy Bones: - Adequate Calcium Intake: Take in foods high in calcium, such as dairy goods, leafy green vegetables, nuts, and seeds. If needed, think about calcium supplements.

- Vitamin D: Follow healthcare professionals' recommendations to ensure adequate vitamin D levels through sun exposure, fortified meals, or supplements.

Weight-bearing activity on a regular basis To strengthen bones, take part in weight-bearing exercises like running, dancing, or weightlifting.

- Drink in moderation and stop smoking: Smoking and excessive alcohol use can have a detrimental effect on bone health.

- Hormonal considerations: To promote bone health throughout menopause, talk to your healthcare professionals about hormone replacement therapy (HRT) or alternative therapies.

- Fall prevention: Take steps to avoid falls by maintaining a clutter-free environment, utilizing assistive equipment when necessary, and making sure your house is properly lit and safe.


4. Diagnosis and screening:

- Dual-energy X-ray absorptiometry (DXA): This bone mineral density test analyzes bone density at key places and aids in determining osteoporosis or determining the likelihood of fracture.

- Speak with your doctor about when and how frequently to get a bone density screening.


5. Osteoporosis Treatment and Management: - Medication: Healthcare professionals may recommend drugs to stop future bone loss or encourage bone production, depending on the severity of the condition and the patient's unique situation.

- Changes in lifestyle: Place a focus on a balanced diet, consistent exercise, quitting smoking, consuming just a small amount of alcohol, and fall prevention techniques.

Supplemental calcium and vitamin D may be advised by medical professionals if food consumption is insufficient to satisfy daily needs.

6. Consistent Follow-Up: - Keep in touch with medical professionals to monitor bone health, assess therapy efficacy, and make appropriate modifications.

Keep in mind that osteoporosis prevention and early treatments are essential for preserving bone health. Adopting a complete strategy that include a balanced diet, frequent exercise, and other healthy lifestyle decisions is crucial. Consult with medical professionals to receive individualized advice based on your unique risk factors and requirements.

# 3

# Mental and Emotional Health

1. Recognizing emotional and mental health

- The total condition of a person's emotional and psychological health is referred to as their emotional and mental well-being.

- It includes traits like emotional fortitude, stress control, self-esteem, and the capacity to overcome obstacles and have a positive viewpoint.

2. Self-Care and Self-Awareness: - Give priority to self-care activities that improve emotional health, such as mindfulness training, participating in hobbies, going outside, and fostering deep connections.

- Develop self-awareness by being aware of your feelings, thoughts, and needs, and then taking initiative to address them.

3. Stress Management: - Develop healthy coping strategies, such as deep breathing exercises, meditation, exercise, journaling, or professional help, to deal with stress.

- To reduce excessive stress, learn to say no when it's necessary and establish appropriate boundaries.

4. Developing Resilience: Resilience is the capacity to overcome adversity and deal with life's difficulties.

- Create a support network, engage in positive thinking, establish achievable objectives, and draw lessons from your history to promote resilience.

5. Seeking assistance: - Ask friends, relatives, or other reliable people for assistance or a sympathetic ear.

- If your mental problems are overwhelming or chronic, think about seeking professional assistance. Counseling, treatment, and advice can be given by mental health specialists.

6. strong Relationships: - Develop and preserve strong connections that support your emotional health.

- Surround yourself with positive influences, encourage open communication, and establish clear limits in your interactions.

7. Mindfulness and Meditation: - Use mindfulness techniques to focus attention on the present moment, lower stress levels, and improve general wellbeing.

- Investigate several meditation practices that fit your tastes, such as loving-kindness meditation, guided meditation, or mindfulness of your breathing.

8. Self-Esteem and Self-Compassion: - Identify your strengths, practice self-compassion, and confront your critical thoughts to create a good self-image.

- Take part in self-esteem-enhancing activities, such as setting attainable objectives, taking care of yourself, and celebrating your successes.

9. Balancing Life's Demands: - Make self-care and relaxation a priority while maintaining your work-life balance and setting reasonable expectations.

- Find places where you may ask for help or delegate tasks to reduce unneeded stress and overwhelm.

10. Emotional Awareness and Expression: By recognizing your feelings and finding appropriate methods to express them, you may improve your emotional wellbeing.

- Take part in emotional expression-promoting activities like journaling, artistic outlets, or chatting to a dependable friend or therapist.

Keep in mind that maintaining your mental and emotional health is a continuous process that calls for your attention, introspection, and proactive actions. A more rewarding and resilient existence can result from putting emotional health care practices into practice. Do not hesitate to contact a specialist if you are having serious or ongoing emotional problems.

## Self-care and emotional intelligence

Our entire health and personal development depend on both emotional intelligence and self-care. Let's investigate how these two ideas are related.

1. Self-Awareness: The first step in developing emotional intelligence is to become aware of and understand our own feelings, needs, and strengths.
   - Self-care fosters self-awareness by encouraging us to check in with ourselves, pay attention to our feelings, and recognize our strengths and opportunities for growth.

2. Emotion Regulation: - Emotional intelligence includes the capacity to control and manage our emotions in a way that prevents them from overwhelming us or having a detrimental influence on our wellbeing.
   - We are given the tools and techniques to control our emotions through self-care activities. Finding emotional equilibrium can be facilitated by engaging in practices like meditation, deep breathing exercises, or hobbies.

3. Empathy and Compassion: - Empathy and compassion are key components of emotional intelligence because they help us better understand and relate to the feelings and experiences of others.
   - Self-care cultivates empathy and compassion by reminding us to treat ourselves with the same respect and love. When we take care of ourselves, we accept our own needs and are kind to ourselves.

4. Boundaries and assertiveness are important components of emotional intelligence because they help us stand up for our demands and make sure they are valued.

- By taking care of ourselves, we have the ability to create and uphold healthy boundaries, to say no when it's appropriate, and to effectively express our needs. It gives us the ability to speak out for ourselves and defend our emotional health.

5. Effective Stress Management: A key component of emotional intelligence is the ability to identify and control stress so that it doesn't compromise our mental and physical well-being.

- Self-care is essential for managing stress. Taking part in relaxing activities, including exercising, practicing mindfulness, or developing a hobby, can help lower stress levels and improve emotional well-being.

6. Self-Reflection and Growth: Emotional intelligence promotes ongoing personal development and self-reflection. It entails asking for criticism, taking experience-based lessons to heart, and making an effort to better oneself.

- Self-care provides chances for introspection and personal development. We may encourage personal growth and boost emotional intelligence by setting aside time for solitude, writing, or participating in pursuits that are consistent with our beliefs and objectives.

7. Resilience: - Emotional intelligence helps people be resilient, which is the capacity to overcome adversity and deal with difficulties.

- Self-care habits help us be resilient by giving us the resources to take care of ourselves when things get tough. Self-care exercises increase our mental and emotional fortitude, assisting us in overcoming obstacles and recovering more quickly.

We lay the groundwork for overall well-being by practicing self-care and developing emotional intelligence. With the help of these two ideas, we can build stronger bonds with others, efficiently control our emotions, and put our own wellbeing first. Greater self-awareness, personal development, and general emotional well-being can result from embracing both emotional intelligence and self-care.

## Stress Reduction Methods

We all encounter stress on a regular basis, and good stress management is essential for general wellbeing. You may include the following stress-reduction methods into your daily routine:

1. Deep Breathing: To trigger the body's relaxation response, do deep breathing exercises. Breathe deeply and slowly, paying attention to each inhalation and exhalation. This aids in calming you down and lowers your heart rate.

2. Physical Activity: Exercise frequently to lower stress and improve mood. Endorphins, which are endogenous mood enhancers, are

released during exercise. Find exercises that you love, such as yoga, dancing, walking, running, or any other activity that meets your interests.

3. Mindfulness and Meditation: Engage in mindfulness exercises like mindful breathing or meditation. Being mindful means paying close attention to the here and now without passing judgment. It can aid in calming down, lowering tension, and boosting self-awareness.

4. Time Management: Time management that is done well may reduce stress brought on by feeling overburdened or having little control over your schedule. Set realistic goals, order things according to importance, and divide them into smaller, more achievable steps. When you can, assign responsibilities to others, and get in the habit of declining time-consuming activities.

5. Healthy Lifestyle: Staying hydrated, getting adequate sleep, and eating a balanced meal can all help you lead a healthy lifestyle. A healthy body is better able to tolerate stress if it is well-fed and well-rested.

6. Social Support: Ask friends, relatives, or a support group for assistance. Discussing your thoughts and worries with others can help you get perspective, encouragement, and useful guidance. You may have a sense of support and less isolation if you share your experiences with reliable people.

7. Relaxation Techniques: Include relaxation methods like progressive muscle relaxation, guided visualization, or relaxing music in your daily routine. Find pastimes that help you relax, such taking a bath, reading a book, or doing something you like.

8. Reduce Stress Triggers: Recognize your personal stressors and take steps to reduce them. Setting boundaries, avoiding or managing stressful situations, or making adjustments to your surroundings that encourage calm and lower stress are all examples of how to do this.

9. Use positive self-talk to counter negative ideas with remarks that are uplifting and upbeat. Instead of obsessing on difficulties, reframe stressful events in a more positive way and concentrate on solutions.

10. Seek Support: Don't be afraid to get professional assistance if stress becomes unbearable or continues in spite of your best efforts. An expert in mental health may offer direction, encouragement, and strategies for stress management.

Remember that finding the tactics that work best for you when it comes to stress management may take some time. Put yourself first and be kind to yourself. Try out several methods and approaches to see which ones work best for you in reducing stress and enhancing your general wellbeing.

**Depression and Anxiety in Women**

Everyone, including women, is susceptible to the frequent mental health illnesses anxiety and depression. An overview of anxiety and depression in women is provided below:

1. Anxiety - Excessive worry, dread, and apprehension, which can interfere with day-to-day activities, are the hallmarks of anxiety disorders.

- Anxiety disorders affect women more frequently than they do males, with hormonal changes, cultural pressures, and life transitions (such pregnancy or menopause) all playing a role in this increased incidence.

2. Depression: Depression is a mental condition marked by lingering melancholy, lack of interest or enjoyment in activities, changes in food or sleep patterns, and trouble focusing. Hormonal changes (such as those that occur during the menstrual cycle, pregnancy, or the postpartum period) may contribute to the fact that women are twice as likely as males to develop depression.

3. Contributing Factors: Biological variations in hormone levels, such as those brought on by the menstrual cycle, pregnancy, and menopause, can affect mood and raise the risk of anxiety and depression.

- Psychosocial Factors: Social constraints, gender expectations, difficulties with job and family obligations, care-giving responsibilities, and trauma or abuse experiences can all contribute to women's anxiety and depression.

- Genetics and Family History: A woman's vulnerability to anxiety or depression may be increased by her family's history of these diseases.

- Life Transitions: Significant events in a woman's life, such as childbirth, motherhood, work changes, or difficulties in a romantic relationship, can cause or aggravate anxiety and sadness.

4. Seeking Assistance: It's crucial to get medical assistance if you're exhibiting signs of anxiety or sadness. They are able to provide a precise diagnosis and suggest the best course of action. Therapy (such cognitive-behavioral therapy or interpersonal therapy) and medicine are also options for treatment, as is a combination of the two. Lifestyle adjustments including consistent exercise, stress reduction, a nutritious diet, and social support can also be helpful.

5. Self-Care Techniques: - Engage in self-care practices that enhance mental health, such as taking up a hobby, using relaxation techniques, spending time with loved ones, and establishing boundaries to give self-care priority.

- Give high priority to healthy lifestyle practices including regular exercise, enough sleep, a balanced diet, and moderate alcohol and drug usage.

- Take part in stress-reduction and emotional-well-being-enhancing activities, such writing, mindfulness, or creative pursuits.

6. Social Support: - Ask friends, family, or support groups for assistance. Speaking with people who have gone through

comparable struggles can help with validation, understanding, and coping mechanisms.

- Consider attending support groups designed especially for women's mental health or getting help from a professional.

Keep in mind that every person has a different experience with anxiety and sadness. It's crucial to exercise self-compassion, be patient with yourself, and ask for assistance when you need it. It is possible to control anxiety and depression and enhance general wellbeing with the correct assistance and care.

*Creating Stable Relationships*

Building wholesome connections is crucial to our general pleasure and well-being. Here are some important guidelines to follow in order to foster good connections, whether they be with potential love partners, family members, friends, or coworkers:

1. Effective communication is the cornerstone of any successful relationship. Be open to learning the viewpoints of others, communicate clearly and honestly, and engage in active listening. Respectful and honest communication builds trust, settles disputes, and improves the relationship.

2. Honesty and Trust: The foundation of a strong relationship is honesty and trust. Be dependable, follow through on your commitments, and uphold your privacy. Encourage open and honest communication while fostering a culture that values honesty.

Although it takes time to develop, trust is essential for the development and sustainability of relationships.

3. Boundaries and Respect: When in a partnership, set and respect personal boundaries. Be clear about your requirements and restrictions, and respect other people's boundaries. Respect each other's independence and uniqueness. Independent living is permitted in healthy partnerships, and each other is supported.

4. Empathy and Understanding: Develop empathy by placing yourself in other people's situations and making an effort to comprehend their viewpoints and emotions. Be understanding, acknowledge their suffering, and be prepared to make concessions. Empathy creates greater understanding and relationships while fortifying bonds.

5. Conflict Resolution: Conflicts and disagreements occur naturally in all relationships. Learn effective conflict-resolution techniques include active listening, expressing emotions in a healthy way, and coming up with solutions that benefit both parties. Avoid personal attacks and concentrate on finding a solution rather than winning the debate.

6. Spend precious time fostering and enhancing connections by engaging in shared activities. Take part in joint pastimes, outings, or other interests that you both like. Create opportunity for deep conversations and bonds by connecting often.

7. Mutual Support and Encouragement: Support and promote one another's aspirations and efforts at personal development. Celebrate one other's accomplishments and support one another emotionally when things are tough. Healthy relationships include helping one other out and working as a team.

8. Flexibility and Adaptability: As situations and people change, relationships need to be flexible and adaptable. Be flexible and willing to make concessions as you seek to connect with one another and satisfy each other's needs. Accept development and progress as one.

9. Healthy Conflict Resolution: In any relationship, disagreements and disputes are inevitable. Learn effective conflict-resolution techniques include active listening, expressing emotions in a healthy way, and coming up with solutions that benefit both parties. Avoid personal attacks and concentrate on finding a solution rather than winning the debate.

10. Self-Care and Personal Wellness: Keep in mind that healthy partnerships start with a healthy relationship with oneself. Set limits, prioritize your well-being, and take part in activities that do the same. You provide your best self to your relationships when you take care of yourself.

All parties involved must put in effort, be patient, and be committed to developing good partnerships. It's crucial to keep in mind that no relationship is flawless and that difficulties and disputes are common. However, you may build solid, significant, and happy relationships with people by putting these concepts into practice and upholding open communication, trust, and respect.

**Coping with abuse and trauma**

The process of overcoming trauma and abuse can be difficult and complicated. It's critical to put your safety and wellbeing first if you have endured trauma or abuse. Here are some broad pointers to assist you:

1. Ensure Safety: If you are in imminent danger or at risk, get assistance from a reliable source or call local law enforcement or abuse or domestic violence hotlines. The first concern is to keep you secure.

2. Seek Support: Speak with a network of friends, family, or experts who can offer moral support and direction. Think about confiding in a therapist, support group, or counselor who has received specialized training in trauma and abuse recovery.

3. Process Your Emotions: Permit yourself to experience and name the feelings you have in relation to the abuse or trauma. It's common to feel a variety of emotions, such as fear, grief, rage, or perplexity. Allow yourself to grieve and process these emotions.

4. Self-Care: Take part in self-care practices that promote your physical, emotional, and mental well. This might include things like

working out, relaxing methods, writing, spending time in nature, and taking part in enjoyable hobbies.

5. Seek Professional Assistance: Take into account consulting with a mental health expert who focuses on trauma and abuse. They can provide you coping mechanisms and methods, like as cognitive-behavioral therapy (CBT), eye movement desensitization and reprocessing (EMDR), or other scientifically proven therapies, to deal with the impacts of trauma.

6. Establish limits: To safeguard yourself from additional harm, set limits that are both obvious and enforceable. Learn to express your wants and limitations assertively, and learn to say no. Embrace your boundaries and surround yourself with supportive individuals.

7. Educate Yourself: To better understand your experiences and emotions, educate yourself on the repercussions of abuse and trauma. This information can empower you and direct you toward constructive coping mechanisms.

8. Develop Self-Compassion: Treat yourself with kindness and compassion as you go through the healing process. Recognize that you are not to fault for what happened and that healing takes time. Develop self-forgiveness and self-compassion.

9. Participate in therapies informed by trauma: Take into account therapies that are designed to deal with the effects of trauma on your

mind and body. You can process and recover from traumatic situations with the aid of these therapies.

10. Safety Planning: If you are still in a hazardous or abusive environment, work with a professional or a domestic violence hotline to develop a safety plan. This plan contains measures you can do to safeguard yourself, such locating safe areas, helpful people, and emergency numbers.

Always keep in mind that everyone's path to recovery is different, so it's crucial to seek out expert advice catered to your particular need. It takes time to recover from trauma and abuse, but with help, understanding, and self-care, you can get there and take back control of                               your                               life.

# 4

# Sexual and Reproductive Health

Introduction: A crucial component of a woman's overall wellbeing is her sexual and reproductive health. Contraception, STIs, menstrual health, and sexual wellbeing are just a few of the issues covered in this chapter's discussion of sexual and reproductive health.

1. Contraception and Family Planning: Covers many forms of contraception, including hormonal (birth control pills, patches, injections), barrier (condoms, diaphragms), intrauterine devices (IUDs), and approaches based on fertility awareness.

- Describes each method's efficiency, application, advantages, and potential drawbacks.

- Emphasizes the value of making educated decisions and speaking with healthcare professionals before selecting a contraceptive technique.

- Examines the idea of family planning and the value of pregnancies being planned in order to protect reproductive autonomy and wellbeing.

2. Sexually Transmitted Infections (STIs): - Gives a general review of the most prevalent STIs, such as the human papillomavirus (HPV), chlamydia, gonorrhea, syphilis, herpes, and HIV/AIDS.

- Stresses the value of safe sexual behaviors, including the use of condoms and routine STI tests.

- Discusses the warning signs, symptoms, and available STI prevention and treatment measures.

- Addresses the stigma attached to STIs and promotes destigmatization and open dialogue.


3. Menstrual Health and Hygiene: Examines the menstrual cycle, including hormonal changes, as well as the associated physical and psychological effects.

- Offers information about period hygiene practices, including how to use and discard menstruation items appropriately, how to maintain good menstrual hygiene, and how to deal with typical monthly difficulties.

- Covers the symptoms, treatment, and effects of menstruation diseases and ailments include polycystic ovarian syndrome (PCOS), premenstrual syndrome (PMS), and dysmenorrhea (painful periods). Promotes understanding of menstruation health as a crucial component of general wellbeing and available treatment choices.


4. Sexual wellbeing and Pleasure: - Promotes honest and uplifting conversations on sexual wellbeing, such as sexual desire, arousal, and pleasure.

- Talks on the value of communication, good relationships, and consent in sexual experiences.

- Offers details on sexual enjoyment, exploring one's impulses, and getting through typical obstacles to sexual gratification.

- Addresses typical worries about sexual function and provides advice on how to get expert assistance when necessary.

5. Reproductive Health and Fertility: - Covers preconception care, prenatal care, and postpartum care, among other reproductive health-related subjects.

- Talks about ovulation monitoring and menstrual cycle awareness for women who are trying to conceive or are intending to.

- Emphasizes the significance of complete reproductive healthcare, which includes routine check-ups, screenings,

In summary, this chapter strives to educate women about their sexual and reproductive health. Women may take control of their sexual and reproductive health by being aware of their options, making educated decisions, and getting the right medical treatment.

**Recognizing Sexual Health**

The term "sexual health" refers to a wide category that includes the social, psychological, and physical health aspects of sexuality. It entails being able to engage in joyful and secure sexual encounters as well as having a positive and respectful perspective on sexuality and romantic relationships. When understanding sexual health, keep the following points in mind:

1. Complete Sexual Education: Promoting sexual health requires that all people have access to accurate and age-appropriate sexual education. Anatomy, reproduction, contraception, STIs, consent, wholesome relationships, and communication techniques should all be covered. Comprehensive sexual education encourages healthy sexual activities and gives people the power to make informed decisions.

2. Consent and Boundaries: An essential component of sexual health is consent. Any sexual action requires the explicit and free consent of all people involved. Healthy sexual relationships must be maintained by respecting and comprehending personal limits. Consent ought to be continuous and revocable at any point.

3. STI Testing and Prevention: It's critical for sexual health to understand how to lower the risk of STIs and take precautions to avoid them. This entails utilizing barrier means of contraception (such condoms), doing routine STI testing, and engaging in safe sex practices. To preserve sexual health and stop future transmission, it is essential to get tested for STIs and get treatment as needed.

4. Reproductive Health: Aspects of reproductive health include contraception, family planning, preconception care, prenatal care, and postpartum care. Sexual health also encompasses reproductive health. It is crucial for people to have access to reproductive healthcare services, such as counseling, testing, and support, in order to be able to make educated decisions about their reproductive options.

5. Building Respectful Relationships and Communication: Sexual health depends on having respectful and healthy relationships. Open communication, faith in one another, trust, and support are examples of this. Maintaining healthy and enjoyable sexual encounters depends on effective communication about sexual wants, limits, and expectations.

6. Sexual Orientation and Gender Identity: It's critical for sexual health to acknowledge and accept the variety of sexual orientations and gender identities. Without stigma or prejudice, everyone has the freedom to express their gender identity and sexual orientation. Promoting inclusive and affirming sexual healthcare involves recognizing and meeting the specific needs of LGBTQ+ people in terms of sexual health.

7. Mental and Emotional Health: Sexual health and mental and emotional health are intertwined. It entails fostering a good sense of one's physical appearance, self-worth, and sexual orientation. For general sexual well-being, it's crucial to address mental health conditions like anxiety, despair, or trauma.

8. Responsible Sexual activity: An important component of sexual health is accepting responsibility for one's sexual activity. This is being conscious of the possible negative effects of sexual activity, such as unexpected pregnancies or STIs, and taking the necessary precautions to avoid them. It also entails respecting other people's limits and rights.

9. Enjoyable and Safe Sexual encounters: Sexual health includes pursuing enjoyable, agreeable, and safe sexual encounters. A meaningful and gratifying sexual life is influenced by one's ability to recognize and respect one's own preferences, wants, and boundaries. Consent, curiosity, and open communication are essential for fostering satisfying sexual experiences.

10. Seeking Support and Resources: It's critical for people to seek support from medical experts, counselors, or sexual health groups if they have worries or inquiries about their sexual health. These sites can offer precise information, direction, and assistance in resolving sexual health issues.

To have meaningful and healthy sexual lives, people need to understand and promote sexual health. It entails information, honest communication, permission, and availability of all available sexual healthcare treatments. People may cultivate healthy attitudes, connections, and sexual experiences by placing a high priority on their sexual health.

## Family Planning and Contraception

Family planning and contraception are crucial components of sexual and reproductive health for both individuals and couples. They provide you the power to make well-informed choices about when to start a family, how far apart to space pregnancies, and how many kids you want. Here is a summary of family planning and contraception:

1. The significance of contraception: The term "contraception" refers to techniques or tools used to avoid becoming pregnant. It gives people and couples the flexibility to decide if and when to start a family, allowing them to organize their lives, pursue their educational and professional ambitions, and preserve their general well-being.

2. Different types of contraceptive techniques exist, each with unique benefits, efficacy, and factors to take into account. Typical techniques include:

- Barrier methods, which physically prevent sperm from accessing the egg, include male and female condoms, diaphragms, and cervical caps.

- Hormonal Techniques: These include contraceptive pills, patches, shots, and hormonal intrauterine devices (IUDs), which employ hormones to suppress ovulation or thicken cervical mucus, preventing conception.

- Long-Acting Reversible Contraceptives (LARCs), which offer reliable contraception over a protracted length of time without needing regular user activity. Examples include hormonal and non-hormonal IUDs and contraceptive implants.

- Emergency contraception: Also referred to as the "morning-after pill," it can be used to avoid pregnancy following unprotected intercourse or the failure of a contraceptive method.

- Fertility Awareness-Based Techniques: These entail monitoring menstrual cycles and spotting fertile and infertile times in order to prevent or prepare for conception.

3. Contraceptive Method Effectiveness: There are a variety of contraceptive techniques available. Condoms, for example, may have a greater failure rate if not used regularly and appropriately, but hormonal implants and IUDs have very low failure rates. To choose the best course of action, it's crucial to examine the efficacy, advantages, and side effects of various techniques with a healthcare professional.

4. Access and Availability: Everyone should have access to and availability of contraceptive techniques. This involves

comprehensive sexual education, free and easy access to contraception, and counseling to help people make educated decisions. The distribution of contraceptive services and information is greatly aided by medical professionals, clinics, and reproductive health groups.

5. Family Planning: Considering pregnancy and the best time to have children requires family planning. It enables individuals and couples to prepare for the resources required to support their children, spacing their pregnancies for better maternal and child health outcomes, and have healthier pregnancies. Family planning encourages sexual and reproductive freedom as well as the health of people, families, and communities.

6. Counseling and assistance: It's crucial to seek out counseling and assistance from medical experts while thinking about contraception and family planning. They can advise on the best strategies depending on each person's needs, preferences, medical background, and future ambitions. Talking about potential adverse effects, use guidelines, and how to transition between techniques if desired are all topics covered in counseling.

7. Shared Decision-Making: Partners should collaborate to decide on family planning and contraception. Communication regarding aspirations, goals, and preferences must be open and honest. With shared decision-making, both spouses take an active role in selecting the best form of contraception for their needs and objectives.

Keep in mind that not every woman is a candidate for every type of contraception. It's crucial to seek the advice of medical specialists when choosing the best contraceptive technique for a given set of circumstances and preferences. Contraceptive techniques are continuously assessed and discussed with healthcare professionals to ensure that they are still appropriate and effective.

**STIs (sex-transmitted infections)**

Infections that are largely spread via sexual activity are called sexually transmitted infections (STIs), commonly referred to as sexually transmitted diseases (STDs). They may be brought on by microbes such as bacteria, viruses, parasites, or others. For prevention, early identification, and appropriate treatment, it is essential to understand STIs. Key details concerning STIs are as follows:

1. Common STIs: There are many different kinds of STIs, such as:

Chlamydia is one of the most prevalent STIs and can affect both men and women. It is brought on by the bacteria Chlamydia trachomatis. Although it frequently shows no symptoms, if left untreated, it can result in catastrophic problems.

- Gonorrhea: This illness of the genitalia, rectum, and throat is brought on by the bacteria Neisseria gonorrhoeae. Discharge, soreness, and discomfort may all be symptoms.

- Syphilis: This disease, which is brought on by the bacteria Treponema pallidum, develops in phases and, if ignored, can result in sores, rashes, and organ damage.

- Human papillomavirus (HPV): A virus that can lead to genital warts and is linked to several cancers, including throat, anal, and cervical cancer.

- Herpes: This condition is brought on by the herpes simplex virus (HSV) and can result in painful blisters or sores in the mouth or genital region. The virus may lay latent in the body for some time before regularly reactivating.

- The acquired immunodeficiency syndrome (AIDS) is brought on by the human immunodeficiency virus (HIV), a viral infection that destroys the immune system. It can be passed from mother to kid through childbirth or nursing, through sexual contact, infected needles, or other means.

- Hepatitis B and C: Viral illnesses that mostly impact the liver and can be spread by intercourse or contact with contaminated blood.

2. Transmission: Sexual acts such as vaginal, anal, and oral sex are the most common ways that STIs are spread. They can be transmitted by contact with contaminated skin or mucous membranes, as well as through contact with infected vaginal, oral, or anal secretions. Some STIs, like HIV, can also be spread by sharing needles or using blood that has been tainted.

3. Prevention: Adopt safe sex habits. STI transmission risk can be decreased by wearing condoms consistently and appropriately.

Condoms should be used throughout all sexual activity, including oral, vaginal, and anal intercourse, from the beginning to the conclusion.

- Vaccination: There are vaccines available for several STIs, including hepatitis B and HPV. Protection from these illnesses may be obtained by vaccination.

Regular STI testing is crucial for early discovery and prompt treatment, particularly if you're sexually active or engaged in high-risk activities.

- Mutual monogamy: Having sex with an uninfected partner while maintaining a mutually monogamous relationship can lower the chance of STI transmission.

- Open communication: To make well-informed decisions and lower the risk of STI transmission, it is crucial to discuss sexual history, STI testing, and utilizing protection with partners.

4. Symptoms and Complications: STIs can cause a variety of symptoms or they can go unnoticed. Genital sores, discharge, itching, pain while urinating, and flu-like symptoms are a few examples of common symptoms. However, certain STIs may not show any symptoms at all. If ignored, STIs can result in consequences such pelvic inflammatory disease, infertility, persistent pain, an elevated risk of HIV transmission, and certain malignancies.

5. Testing and Treatment: There are many different ways to test for STIs, including blood tests, urine tests, swabs, and physical examinations. Depending on the individual STI, there are many treatment approaches that may

Infertility and Fertility

Important facets of women's reproductive health include fertility and infertility. Let's examine the following subjects:

1. Fertility: The capacity to conceive and carry a healthy pregnancy is referred to as fertility. Age, general health, hormone balance, and reproductive anatomy are some of the variables that affect it. Women are most fertile throughout their reproductive years, which normally begin with the commencement of menstruation (menarche) and terminate with menopause. However, fertility can vary from person to person, and it's crucial to remember that fertility reduces with age, especially beyond the age of 35.

2. Recognizing the Menstrual Cycle: The menstrual cycle is important for fertility. The body gets ready for pregnancy once a month. The cycle is controlled by hormones, chiefly estrogen and progesterone, and it involves the release of an egg (ovulation) from the ovaries. A pregnancy could result from the egg implanting in the uterus after being fertilized by sperm.

3. Fertility-Related Factors: A number of variables might affect a woman's fertility, including:

- Age: Fertility decreases with age, especially beyond the age of 35, as a result of a loss in egg quantity and quality.

- Medical issues: A number of health issues, including polycystic ovarian syndrome (PCOS), endometriosis, and reproductive issues, can have an impact on fertility.

- Lifestyle elements: Things like smoking, binge drinking, drug use, obesity, and poor nutrition might have an impact on fertility.

- Hormonal imbalances: Irregular menstrual cycles and thyroid problems are two conditions that might affect fertility.

- Pelvic infections: Reproductive system infections can harm and scar the organs, which can reduce fertility.

- Stress and emotional variables: Long-term stress and emotional issues might affect fertility and the hormonal balance.

4. Infertility: Infertility is the inability to conceive after attempting for a predetermined amount of time (usually one year for women under 35 or six months for women over 35) or the inability to carry a pregnancy to term. Ovulation problems, blocked Fallopian tubes, hormone imbalances, uterine abnormalities, and male factor infertility are only a few of the causes of infertility. It's crucial to keep in mind that both men and women might experience infertility.

5. Seeking Assistance for Infertility: If you're experiencing trouble conceiving, it's best to seek assistance from a healthcare provider with expertise in reproductive health. They can do tests, assess your

medical history, and offer advice on possible infertility causes. Infertility can be treated with fertility drugs, surgery, assisted reproductive technology (such in vitro fertilization), or by taking care of underlying health issues.

6. Emotional Support: Coping with reproductive issues emotionally can be difficult. It's crucial to ask your partner, close friends, or support groups for emotional assistance. Additionally helpful in handling the emotional side of infertility is counseling or therapy.

7. Fertility Preservation: Options like egg freezing or embryo freezing can be taken into consideration by women who prefer to protect their fertility for a variety of reasons, including medical treatments that can compromise fertility or postponing motherhood. These techniques enable the storage of eggs or embryos for the future.

Keep in mind that every person's road to becoming pregnant is different, and there are many tools and solutions available to assist individuals and couples as they deal with fertility and infertility issues. Understanding and taking care of fertility issues may be facilitated by seeking assistance, being knowledgeable, and collaborating with healthcare specialists.

*Prenatal Health and Pregnancy Care*

A woman's life is transformed and fascinating throughout pregnancy. For the sake of both you and your unborn child, it is imperative that you take good care of your health throughout pregnancy. The following are significant elements of prenatal care:

1. Prenatal Healthcare Provider: Early in pregnancy, it's crucial to choose a healthcare professional who specializes in prenatal care, such as an obstetrician, midwife, or family doctor. You may get the right medical advice, follow the development of your pregnancy, and handle any worries or issues with frequent prenatal checkups.

2. Healthy Lifestyle: It's crucial to keep up a healthy lifestyle when pregnant. Focus on the following significant factors:
   - Nutrition: Consume a variety of fruits, vegetables, whole grains, lean proteins, and dairy products as part of a balanced diet. Avoid alcohol, under cooked or raw meals, excessive caffeine, and some seafood that contain high mercury levels.
   - Weight management: Follow your healthcare provider's advice on the optimal amount of weight gain throughout pregnancy. Gaining too much or too little weight can have an effect on both your health and the development of the unborn child.
   - Physical exercise: Take part in routine, safe, pregnancy-safe physical activity. If you're unsure about the right workouts to do, speak with your healthcare professional.
   - Prenatal vitamins: Follow your doctor's advice and take the prenatal vitamins, which often contain folic acid, iron, and other vital minerals.

3. Prenatal Tests and Screenings: To monitor your health and determine the wellbeing of your unborn child, your healthcare

practitioner may suggest a number of prenatal tests and screenings. These might include of blood testing, ultrasounds, genetic screenings, and examinations for preeclampsia or gestational diabetes, among other things.

4. Managing Symptoms and Discomforts: The discomforts of pregnancy might include nausea, exhaustion, back pain, and mood changes. Consult your healthcare professional about any worries or symptoms so they can advise you on how to safely manage these discomforts.

5. prenatal Education and Preparedness: To learn more about pregnancy, labor, nursing, infant care, and parenting, think about enrolling in prenatal classes or educational programs. You may learn useful knowledge from these programs, which will make you feel more equipped for the adventure ahead.

6. Emotional and Mental Well-being: Hormonal shifts and a wide variety of emotions are common throughout pregnancy. You should give your emotional health top priority. Ask your partner, family, and friends for support, and if necessary, think about joining support groups or going to counseling.

7. Avoiding Harmful drugs: It's important to stay away from drugs that can damage both you and your unborn child while you're pregnant. These include using tobacco products, alcohol, illegal substances, certain prescriptions, and exposure to pollutants in the environment.

8. Rest and Sleep: Pregnancy requires a sufficient amount of rest and sleep. Pay attention to what your body needs and put getting enough rest and relaxation first.

9. Birth Plan: Think about writing down your choices for labor, delivery, and postpartum care in a birth plan. Make sure your healthcare provider is aware of your desires by talking to them about it.

10. Postpartum Care: Keep in mind that pregnancy care continues throughout the time following delivery. Create a postpartum care plan that includes assistance with nursing, healing, and mental health.

Throughout your pregnancy, always seek the counsel and direction of your healthcare professional. Every pregnancy is different, and they will provide you the best advice depending on your particular situation.

**Care after delivery and mental health**

The time immediately following childbirth is referred to as the postpartum phase, during which a woman's body experiences physical and hormonal changes while she acclimates to the duties of caring for her infant. Important factors in supporting the wellbeing of both the mother and the child are postpartum care and mental health. Important factors for postpartum care and mental health include the following:

1. Physical healing: Following labor, the postpartum phase comprises physical healing. Here are some details to pay attention to:

- Rest and sleep: Getting enough rest and sleep is crucial for healing and recharging the body's energy reserves. Take advantage of the time your baby spends sleeping to rest.

    - Follow your healthcare provider's instructions for perineal care and wound healing if you had perineal tears or gave birth through cesarean section.

    - Pain management: Talk to your healthcare practitioner about any pain or discomfort you are experiencing so they can offer the best pain management techniques.

    - Postpartum bleeding: After giving delivery, some vaginal bleeding (lochia) is normal. When using sanitary pads, follow the directions carefully, and let your healthcare professional know if bleeding becomes heavy or worrisome.

    - Breast care: If you are nursing, look after your breasts by making sure the latch is correct, using nipple creams if necessary, and getting help if you are having any difficulties.

2. Mental health and emotional stability:

There might be a wide range of feelings and adaptations throughout the postpartum period. Key factors to keep in mind for preserving mental health are as follows:

- Baby blues: Mood swings, irritability, and melancholy, sometimes known as the baby blues, are frequently experienced by new moms. Over the course of a few weeks, these symptoms often go away on their own.

Depression after childbirth (PPD): PPD is a more significant disorder that calls for medical intervention. Seek treatment from your healthcare professional right away if you frequently feel depressed, anxious, bored, have trouble bonding with your child, or have suicidal thoughts.

- Postpartum anxiety: During this time, some women may feel excessive concern, panic attacks, or obsessive-compulsive behaviors. If you are having these symptoms, see your healthcare physician.

- Ask for help: To get emotional support, connect with your spouse, your family, and your friends. joining support groups, both in-person and online,can also offer a helpful network of people who understand and who can give advice.

- Self-care: Give yourself the time and attention they need to help you unwind, relax, and preserve your mental health. This could entail taking pauses, participating in hobbies, engaging in mindfulness or meditation, and, as needed, getting assistance with domestic chores.

3. Postpartum Check-ups: Go to your prearranged postpartum check-ups with your doctor to monitor your healing, discuss any worries, and get advice on using contraception, nursing, and getting back to your normal activities.

4. Seeking Assistance: Do not hesitate to seek assistance if you are having problems or worries about postpartum care or your mental health. Your healthcare practitioner can provide suitable resources, referrals, or treatment alternatives and is available to help you.

Remember that both you and your baby need postpartum care and mental health support. Self-care encourages a healthy start to motherhood and enables you to provide for your infant more effectively. Be upfront about your emotions, reach out for support, and, if necessary, seek professional assistance. Resources are available to support you throughout this crucial changeover phase, so you are not alone.

# 5

# Hormone balance

The general health and wellbeing of a woman is significantly influenced by hormones. They control a number of bodily functions, such as the menstrual cycle, fertility, mood, metabolism, and more. For preserving balance and addressing any potential imbalances or illnesses, it is essential to comprehend hormonal health. We will examine significant facets of hormonal health in this chapter, including:

1. The Functions of Hormones:

- Estrogen: Estrogen is a major female sex hormone that controls secondary sexual traits, the menstrual cycle, and the growth and development of the reproductive system.

- Progesterone: Progesterone is a vital female hormone that helps to promote pregnancy, regulate the menstrual cycle, and get the body ready for childbirth.

- Testosterone: Despite being generally associated with men, testosterone is also found in women and supports a variety of bodily functions, including desire, energy, muscular mass, and bone density.

2. Hormonal Imbalances: Stress, lifestyle choices, underlying medical issues, or aging-related changes are just a few causes of hormonal imbalances. Typical hormonal abnormalities in women include the following:

- Polycystic Ovary Syndrome (PCOS): PCOS is a hormonal condition marked by an imbalance of the hormones testosterone, progesterone, and estrogen. It can cause symptoms such as irregular periods, infertility problems, weight gain, and others.

- Thyroid Disorders: Illnesses such as hypothyroidism or hyperthyroidism can impair the thyroid gland's normal operation, altering hormone synthesis and metabolism.

Menopause is a stage of a woman's life when her ovaries stop producing eggs and her menstrual cycles halt. Hormonal changes, such as a drop in estrogen and progesterone levels, characterize this transition.

Premenstrual syndrome (PMS) is the term used to describe a variety of physical and mental symptoms that appear prior to menstruation and are frequently brought on by hormonal changes.

3. Managing Hormonal Health: It's crucial to keep your hormones in check if you want to be healthy all around. Here are several methods to promote hormonal balance:

- Leading a healthy lifestyle: A balanced diet, consistent exercise, sufficient sleep, and stress-reduction practices can all help to maintain hormonal balance.

- Hormone replacement treatment (HRT): In some circumstances, HRT may be advised to treat symptoms brought on by hormonal imbalances, such as menopause.

- Medication: To control hormone levels and treat problems like PCOS or irregular periods, medication or hormonal contraceptives may be administered.

- Natural remedies: Acupuncture, herbal supplements, and certain dietary adjustments are a few examples of natural treatments that some women use to treat hormone imbalances. Before attempting any new treatments, it is crucial to speak with a healthcare provider.

4. Seeking Professional Assistance: It's critical to speak with a healthcare practitioner if you think you may have a hormone imbalance or encounter symptoms that might point to one. They can do tests, assess your symptoms, and suggest the best actions or therapies to get your hormones back in balance.

5. Regular Health Checkups: Monitoring and controlling hormonal health requires regular health checks, which should include evaluations of hormone levels. Consult your healthcare practitioner if you have any questions or notice any changes in your menstrual cycle, mood, level of energy, or general well-being.

It's critical to comprehend your hormonal health and take care of it if you want to retain general health and wellbeing as a lady. You can support your body's natural processes and encourage hormonal balance by leading a healthy lifestyle, remaining informed, and getting expert assistance when necessary. Keep in mind that every woman's road to hormonal health is different, and what works for one woman may not work for another. Together, you and your healthcare practitioner may create a unique plan that caters to your unique requirements.

**Hormonal disorders and imbalances**

When there are interruptions or anomalies in the production, regulation, or functioning of hormones in the body, hormonal imbalances and diseases may result. These abnormalities can have an impact on a woman's reproductive system, metabolism, emotions, and general well-being, among other elements of her health. The following list of typical hormonal imbalances and conditions that affect women includes:

1. Polycystic Ovarian Syndrome (PCOS): PCOS is a hormonal condition marked by an imbalance of the hormones testosterone, progesterone, and estrogen. Small cysts can form in the ovaries as a result, which can cause symptoms including irregular or skipped periods, increased hair growth, acne, weight gain, and problems with conception.

2. Thyroid problems: Thyroid problems, such hypothyroidism (an under-active thyroid) or hyperthyroidism (an overactive thyroid), can impair the thyroid gland's regular operation, which results in the production of hormones that control metabolism. Fatigue, weight fluctuations, mood swings, hair loss, and irregular menstruation cycles can all be signs of thyroid issues.

3. Menopause: A woman experiences menopause naturally, which is characterized by a drop in estrogen and progesterone levels when her ovaries cease producing eggs. It usually strikes between the ages of 45 and 55 and is characterized by symptoms including hot flashes, nocturnal sweats, mood swings, vaginal dryness, and changes in menstruation cycles.

4. Premenstrual Syndrome (PMS): PMS is the name given to a collection of mental and physical symptoms that appear a few days or weeks before a period. It is thought that hormonal changes, notably variations in estrogen and progesterone levels, are a factor in PMS symptoms. Bloating, breast discomfort, mood fluctuations, irritability, exhaustion, and food cravings are typical symptoms.

5. Endometriosis: In endometriosis, the tissue that ordinarily lines the uterus develops outside the uterus, commonly on the ovaries, Fallopian tubes, or pelvic lining. The illness is impacted by hormonal changes and can result in symptoms including pelvic discomfort, painful sexual activity, heavy menstrual cycles, and infertility.

6. Hyperandrogenism: Women who have hyperandrogenism often have high amounts of androgens (male hormones). It may result in symptoms including male pattern baldness, acne, and excessive hair growth (hirsutism).

7. Adrenal Disorders: Conditions like Cushing's disease and adrenal insufficiency that affect the adrenal glands can impair the synthesis

of hormones like cortisol and aldosterone. Numerous symptoms, including as weight gain, exhaustion, mood swings, and irregular menstrual cycles, can be brought on by these illnesses.

It is crucial to keep in mind that the origins, signs, and severity of hormonal imbalances and illnesses might vary. It is advised to speak with a healthcare professional who can assess your symptoms, carry out the required tests, and offer suitable treatment choices if you suspect a hormone imbalance or are concerned about your hormonal health. Depending on the problem at hand and its underlying causes, treatment may entail a combination of lifestyle modifications, drugs, hormone replacement therapy, and other measures.

## (PCOS) Polycystic Ovary Syndrome

Women of reproductive age frequently have PCOS, a hormonal condition known as polycystic ovary syndrome. Hormonal dysregulation, particularly increased androgen (male hormone) levels in the body, characterize it. A woman's reproductive system may be affected by PCOS for a while and experience a range of symptoms and metabolic well-being. These are some crucial details concerning PCOS:

1. Symptoms: Women can have several PCOS symptoms, which can range from:

- Infrequent, irregular, or nonexistent menstrual cycles: PCOS can result in irregular, protracted, or absent menstrual cycles.

- Excessive hair growth (hirsutism): Women with PCOS may suffer excessive hair growth on their faces, chests, backs, or other parts of their bodies as a result of elevated testosterone levels.

- Acne: Hormonal imbalances can cause acne outbreaks, especially on the lower face, chin, and jawline.

- Weight gain: Many PCOS sufferers battle with weight gain or find it challenging to shed pounds, especially around the midsection.

- Hair loss: PCOS has been linked to hair thinning or scalp hair loss.

- Skin changes: The skin may darken in certain places, such as the wrinkles around the neck, beneath the breasts, or in the crotch.

- Difficulty becoming pregnant: PCOS can affect fertility because of irregular or absent ovulation.


2. Causes: While the precise etiology of PCOS is unknown, it is thought to be a result of a mix of hereditary and environmental factors. PCOS is frequently linked to insulin resistance, which impairs the body's capacity to use insulin efficiently. Hormonal imbalances can result from elevated insulin levels because they encourage the ovaries to create more androgens.


3. Diagnosis: A medical history evaluation, physical examination, and laboratory testing are used to diagnose PCOS. The presence of two out of the three essential symptoms—irregular or nonexistent menstrual cycles, clinical or biochemical indications of elevated

testosterone levels, and ultrasound confirmation of polycystic ovaries—is often required for a diagnosis to be made.

4. Management and Treatment: The management of PCOS focuses on treating specific symptoms and reducing the condition's long-term health hazards. Treatment choices might be:

- Lifestyle adjustments: Adopting a healthy lifestyle with regular exercise, a balanced diet, and weight control can help increase insulin sensitivity and control hormone levels.

- Medication: Different drugs, including hormonal contraceptives (to control menstrual cycles), anti-androgen medications (to minimize excessive hair growth and acne), and medications to manage insulin resistance, may be recommended depending on the symptoms and treatment objectives.

- Fertility treatments: Ovulation induction or assisted reproductive technologies may be helpful for women with PCOS who are having trouble becoming pregnant.

Regular checkups and monitoring are crucial to managing symptoms, evaluating the efficacy of medication, and keeping an eye on long-term health concerns related to PCOS, such as diabetes, cardiovascular disease, and endometrial cancer.

Working closely with medical professionals who specialize in reproductive and hormonal health is crucial for women with PCOS. They can offer direction, tailored treatment programs, and continuous support to help you manage the disease and enhance your general wellbeing.

**Causes, Symptoms, and Treatment of Endometriosis**

Endometriosis is a persistent disorder in which the endometrium, the tissue that typically lines the inside of the uterus, develops on structures other than the uterus, most frequently the ovaries, Fallopian tubes, and tissues lining the pelvis. Pain, inflammation, and other issues might result from this displaced endometrial tissue. An summary of the causes, symptoms, and available therapies for endometriosis may be found here:

1. Causes: Although the precise etiology of endometriosis is unknown, various suggestions have been put forth, including:

- Retrograde menstruation: According to this idea, endometrial cells from menstrual blood travel retrogradely down the Fallopian tubes and into the pelvic cavity, where they implant and develop.

- Hormonal factors: Imbalances in estrogen and progesterone, in particular, may be responsible for the onset and progression of endometriosis.

- Immune system dysfunction: An immune system that is not functioning properly may be unable to identify and get rid of the endometrial tissue that has grown in the wrong area, causing inflammation.

2. Symptoms: The symptoms of endometriosis can fluctuate widely in intensity from woman to woman. Typical signs include:

- Pelvic discomfort: A defining sign of endometriosis is chronic, perhaps severe pelvic pain. The discomfort may come on before and during a period, during a sexual encounter, or even during bowel or urinal motions.

- Irregular menstrual cycles: Endometriosis can cause severe or protracted menstrual bleeding, irregular menstrual cycles, or spotting in between periods in affected women.

- Painful intercourse: A typical symptom is intense discomfort during or after sexual intercourse.

- Infertility: Endometriosis can impair fertility by impacting the operation of the uterus, ovaries, and Fallopian tubes.

- Digestive issues: Particularly during menstruation, some women may develop digestive issues including bloating, diarrhea, constipation, or nausea.

3. Diagnosis: The diagnosis of endometriosis often entails the evaluation of the patient's medical history, a physical exam, imaging tests, and occasionally laparoscopic surgery to see and sample the endometrial implants for confirmation.

4. therapy: The goal of endometriosis therapy is to control symptoms, stop the spread of the condition, and enhance quality of life. Options for treatment include:

- Painkillers: Nonsteroidal anti-inflammatory medicines (NSAIDs), which are available over-the-counter, can help control pain and inflammation.

- Hormonal therapy: Hormonal treatments, including as progestins, gonadotropin-releasing hormone (GnRH) agonists, and aromatase inhibitors, can help control hormonal fluctuations and lessen the development and activity of endometrial tissue.

- Surgery: Endometrial implants and scar tissue are frequently removed or destroyed during laparoscopic surgery. A hysterectomy, or removal of the uterus, may be advised in extreme instances.

- Fertility treatments: In vitro fertilization (IVF) and other assisted reproductive technologies may be used to treat infertility in women who have endometriosis.

Working closely with medical professionals who specialize in the issue is crucial for women with endometriosis who have been identified or suspected of having the disease. They may help with the physical and psychological effects of having endometriosis by offering the right kinds of therapies, pain-relieving techniques, and emotional support.

*Women's Thyroid Disorders*

According to some estimates, women are five to eight times more likely than males to experience thyroid issues. Thyroid abnormalities are widespread in women. The thyroid is a little gland in the front of the neck that regulates metabolism and makes hormones that affect many different biological processes. The kinds, causes, symptoms, and treatments of thyroid problems in women are listed below:

1.Types of Thyroid Conditions

- Hypothyroidism: This disorder is brought on by insufficient thyroid hormone production. Common reasons include the autoimmune condition Hashimoto's thyroiditis, thyroid surgery, radiation treatment, and certain drugs. Constipation, depression, cold sensitivity, lethargy, and weight gain are some signs of hypothyroidism.

- Hyperthyroidism: The reverse of hypothyroidism, hyperthyroidism is characterized by excessive thyroid hormone production. The autoimmune disorder Graves' disease is the most frequent cause of hyperthyroidism. Weight loss, an accelerated pulse, increased perspiration, anxiety, irritability, and tremors are some of the signs of hyperthyroidism.

- Thyroid nodules: In the thyroid gland, thyroid nodules are abnormal growths or lumps. Although benign nodules constitute the majority, some can be malignant. Thyroid nodules can be found by physical examinations or imaging studies even though they frequently do not show any symptoms.

2. Causes of Thyroid abnormalities: - Autoimmune illnesses: The most frequent causes of thyroid abnormalities are autoimmune illnesses including Hashimoto's thyroiditis and Graves' disease. In

these circumstances, the thyroid gland is erroneously attacked by the immune system, causing inflammation and malfunction.

- Iodine deficiency: A lack of iodine in the diet can hinder the thyroid's ability to produce hormones, which can lead to hypothyroidism. Iodine insufficiency is uncommon in areas where salt and other dietary sources are iodized.

- hereditary considerations: Some hereditary factors can make thyroid diseases more likely to occur.

- Other factors: Stress, pregnancy, certain drugs, radiation exposure, and prior thyroid surgery are all potential causes or influences of some thyroid problems.


3. Diagnosis and Treatment: - Diagnosis: Thyroid problems are frequently identified by blood tests that check levels of thyroid hormones (such as TSH, T3, and T4) and antibodies linked to autoimmune thyroid illnesses. A thyroid gland imaging test, such as an ultrasound or radioactive iodine uptake, may also be performed to measure the thyroid's size and functionality.

- Treatment: The kind and severity of the thyroid problem will determine the available treatments. Commonly used therapies include:

- Hypothyroidism: To restore normal hormone levels, hypothyroidism is often treated with synthetic thyroid hormone replacement therapy (levothyroxine).

- Hyperthyroidism: There are several ways to treat this condition, including surgery to remove the thyroid gland, radioactive iodine therapy to destroy a portion of the thyroid gland, and medication to lower thyroid hormone production (such as antithyroid medications).

- Thyroid nodules: The size, features, and likelihood of malignancy of thyroid nodules determine how they should be treated. Options include waiting it out, taking medicine to make nodules smaller, or removing the thyroid gland entirely surgically.

Regular follow-up visits with medical professionals are crucial for women with thyroid problems to check hormone levels, make necessary medication adjustments, and address any lingering issues. The majority of women with thyroid issues may live healthy, productive lives with the right diagnosis and treatment.

# 6

# Screening and Preventative Medicine

Maintaining women's health and avoiding numerous illnesses requires preventive treatment and routine tests. This chapter focuses on the significance of screening procedures and preventative care that women should think about. These are some of the main subjects this chapter covers:

1. Well-Woman examinations: Well-woman examinations are regular checkups with a preventative care and general health focus on women. A review of the patient's medical history, a physical examination, a breast exam, a pelvic exam, and conversations about reproductive health, contraception, and lifestyle issues are often included in these examinations. Healthcare professionals have the chance to evaluate overall health, spot early indications of disorders, and offer pertinent advice and suggestions during well-woman checks.

2. Vaccinations: Vaccinations are essential in the fight against infectious illnesses. Key immunizations for women include the following:

Human papillomavirus (HPV) vaccine: Provides defense against certain strains of HPV that have been linked to malignancies including cervical cancer.

- Influenza vaccine: Annually advised for seasonal influenza protection.

- Tetanus, diphtheria, and pertussis (Tdap) vaccine: Guards against whooping cough, tetanus, and diphtheria.

- The MMR vaccination is crucial for immunization against measles, mumps, and rubella, especially for women who are contemplating pregnancy.

3. Cervical cancer screening: Early identification and prevention of cervical cancer depend on cervical cancer screening. The Pap test, which involves taking cells from the cervix to check for anomalies, is the main screening method. The Pap test and HPV tests may occasionally be combined. Regular cervical cancer screenings can find early-stage cervical cancer or precancerous alterations, enabling prompt intervention and treatment.

4. Breast Cancer Screening: Breast cancer screening seeks to find the disease when it's still treatable and at an early stage. Typical screening techniques include:

- Mammography: Breast imaging with X-rays to look for changes or anomalies.

- Clinical breast examination: A healthcare professional's physical examination of the breasts.

- Breast self-examination: Consistently inspecting your breasts to look for any changes or anomalies.

5. Osteoporosis Screening: The condition osteoporosis is characterized by decreased bone density and an elevated risk of fractures. Bone mineral density (BMD) testing is a component of osteoporosis screening and is frequently carried out using dual-energy X-ray absorptiometry (DXA). Early diagnosis of osteoporosis enables effective therapies, such as dietary changes, calcium and vitamin D supplements, and medication, to stop additional bone loss and lower the risk of fracture.

6. Additional Screenings: Additional screenings and preventative measures that are pertinent to women's health may also be covered in this chapter. These include tests for STIs, cholesterol, blood pressure, diabetes, and certain malignancies (such as colorectal cancer). Discussions on dietary changes, exercise, and lifestyle adjustments as preventive measures may also be addressed.

This chapter strives to encourage women to take control of their health and make educated decisions to preserve their well-being and avoid illnesses by highlighting the value of preventative care and screenings. The early identification, efficient management, and improved results for numerous health disorders may be considerably aided by routine checkups and screenings, as well as living a healthy lifestyle.

## Breast Cancer and Breast Health

Understanding breast cancer is essential for early identification and successful treatment. Breast health is a significant component of women's overall wellbeing. Breast health and breast cancer are the main topics of this chapter, which also discusses breast anatomy, breast self-examination, breast cancer risk factors, screening, and treatment choices. The following are some major subjects that this chapter may touch on:

1. Breast Anatomy and Physiology: In this part, the anatomy and physiology of the breast are briefly discussed, along with an explanation of the various breast structures, including glandular tissue, lobes, ducts, and lymph nodes. Recognizing changes and abnormalities requires knowledge of the typical breast's structure and function.

2. Breast Self-Examination (BSE): Women can use this approach to get to know their breasts and find out if there are any changes or anomalies. The chapter may include a step-by-step procedure for

doing BSE and stress the value of routine self-examination as a method of early detection. It's crucial to remember that BSE recommendations have changed over time, so the most recent suggestions might not be the best ones.

3. Breast Cancer chance variables: This section examines the numerous variables that might raise a woman's chance of getting breast cancer. Age, a family history of breast cancer, genetic mutations like BRCA1 and BRCA2, hormonal factors like early menstruation, late menopause, and hormone replacement therapy, lifestyle factors like alcohol use and obesity, and exposure to specific hormones or chemicals are just a few of the risk factors that may be present. Women may take preventative measures and make educated decisions about their health by being aware of these risk factors.

4. Breast Cancer Screening: Breast cancer screening works to find the disease early on, even before symptoms emerge. Various screening techniques, including mammography, clinical breast examination, and breast self-examination, may be covered in this chapter. The advantages and disadvantages of each screening technique may be highlighted, along with the suggested screening protocols depending on age and risk factors.

5. Breast Cancer Diagnosis and Staging: This section describes the diagnosis and staging of breast cancer, which often entails a biopsy to examine breast tissue and imaging tests (mammography, ultrasound, MRI). It may also clarify the significance of breast

cancer staging, which establishes the degree of disease spread and aids in determining the best course of therapy.

6. Treatment Options: The chapter gives a general review of the many breast cancer treatments, such as surgery (mastectomy or breast-conserving surgery), radiation therapy, chemo, targeted therapy, and hormone therapy. Depending on the stage and features of the cancer, it could go through the objectives of each treatment strategy, any possible adverse effects, and the significance of creating tailored treatment regimens.

7. Breast cancer Survivorship and Support: These two aspects of the breast cancer experience are crucial. This section may examine challenges related to survival, including as managing long-term side effects and preserving general wellbeing. The various resources for help, such as support groups, therapy, and survivorship programs, may also be highlighted.

This chapter seeks to empower women with information about their breast health, promote early detection, encourage routine screenings, and offer advise on treatment options as well as support before, during, and after a breast cancer diagnosis.

**Pap tests and cervical health**

emphasizes the necessity of routine Pap screenings in the early diagnosis of cervical abnormalities and cervical cancer and the importance of cervical wellness. The structure of the cervix, the function of the human papillomavirus (HPV), the use of Pap smears, and the value of routine screening are just a few of the topics covered in this chapter on cervical health. The following are some major subjects that this chapter may touch on:

1. Cervical Anatomy and Physiology: In this part, the anatomy and physiology of the cervix are briefly discussed, along with the cervix's location, structure, and function in the female reproductive system. Understanding the function of Pap smears and cervical health requires a fundamental understanding of the cervix's architecture.

2. Human Papillomavirus (HPV): The chapter may include HPV's impact on cervical health as well as the emergence of abnormalities and cancer of the cervical region. It could discuss the various HPV strains, how they spread, and the connection between high-risk HPV infections and cervical cancer.

3. Pap Smear Procedure and Purpose: This section describes how Pap smears are performed and how they are used to look for precancerous or cancerous cells as well as early indications of cervical abnormalities. The procedure may be described in depth, including sample collection methods such utilizing a tiny brush or spatula to gather cells from the cervix and the significance of a precise and high-quality sample.

4. Screening recommendations and Frequency: The chapter may go through the suggested Pap smear recommendations, including the

recommended age to start screening, the suggested frequency of screening, and when to quit screening. It could address the discrepancies in recommendations based on elements including age, risk factors, and the outcomes of earlier screenings.

5. Interpreting Pap Smear Results: This section discusses the various classifications and results that can be obtained from a Pap smear, such as normal results, abnormal results that may indicate precancerous or cancerous changes, and the importance of follow-up testing and management based on the results.

6. HPV Immunization: As a preventative measure for cervical health, the chapter may discuss HPV vaccination. It could go through the advantages of HPV vaccine, the recommended age for vaccination, and how it helps lower the risk of cervical cancer and HPV-related problems.

7. Cervical Cancer Treatment and Prevention: In this part, the various cervical cancer treatments—including surgery, radiation therapy, chemotherapy, and targeted therapy—may be briefly discussed. The significance of early diagnosis through routine Pap screenings as a preventative technique to detect cervical abnormalities before they develop into cancer may also be emphasized.

This chapter strives to increase knowledge of cervical cancer prevention, empower women to prioritize their cervical health, and persuade them to go through prescribed screenings for early detection and intervention. It does this by emphasising the importance of cervical health and routine Pap smears.

*Uterine and Ovarian Health*

provides crucial details on the anatomy, function, prevalent health problems, and preventative actions connected to the ovary and the uterus, with a focus on ovarian and uterine health. The following are some major subjects that this chapter may touch on:

1. Anatomy and Function of the Ovaries: This section gives a general description of the ovaries and explains where they are located, how they are built, and what their main purposes are. The development of eggs (oocytes) and the release of the hormones (estrogen and progesterone) that are essential for the menstrual cycle and fertility may be covered.

2. Common Ovarian Health Issues: The chapter could discuss common conditions that might have an impact on the ovaries, including ovarian cysts, polycystic ovary syndrome (PCOS), benign and malignant ovarian tumors, and ovarian cancer. It could include details about these disorders' causes, symptoms, diagnostic techniques, and potential treatments.

3. Anatomy and Function of the Uterus: In this part, the uterus (also known as the womb) is described, along with its anatomy and role in the reproductive system. The uterus' function in maintaining

pregnancy, the menstrual cycle, and the changes that take place after birthing may all be covered.

4. Common Uterine Health Issues: The chapter can discuss common conditions that can affect the uterus, including uterine polyps, uterine cancer, endometriosis, and uterine fibroids (noncancerous growths outside the uterus). It could include details about these disorders' causes, symptoms, diagnostic techniques, and potential treatments.

5. Reproductive Health and Fertility: This section may cover how fertility and reproductive capacity may be impacted by the condition of the ovaries and uterus. Topics including fertility assessment, fertility-influencing variables, and assisted reproductive technologies (ART) like in vitro fertilization (IVF) may be covered. It could also cover lifestyle elements that might affect reproductive health, such diet, exercise, and stress management.

6. Preventive Measures and Self-Care: To preserve ovarian and uterine health, the chapter may stress the significance of preventive measures and self-care activities. It might include advice on lifestyle choices that support reproductive health, such eating healthily, engaging in safe sex, and limiting exposure to noxious drugs. It could also emphasize the value of routine gynecological examinations, screening exams (such Pap smears and pelvic exams), and early identification of potential problems.

This chapter's detailed discussion of ovarian and uterine health seeks to inform women on the significance of these reproductive organs, frequent health problems that may occur, and preventative methods to advance their wellbeing. Early identification, prompt action, and proper medical treatment may all be aided by knowledge of the anatomy, symptom recognition, and seeking out the right care.

**Health Screenings and Regular Checkups**

emphasizes the value of routine medical exams and screenings for women's general health and wellbeing. It places a strong emphasis on the value of preventative care, early identification of possible health concerns, and the assistance that medical professionals may provide to women in preserving their health. The following are some major subjects that this chapter may touch on:

1. Gaining an Understanding of Preventive Care: This part gives a general overview of preventive care and explains why it is essential for preserving good health. It could clarify the idea of preventative care, which includes regular checkups, immunizations, screenings, and alterations to one's lifestyle that might aid in preventing or detecting health concerns at an early stage.

2. Primary Care Visits: The chapter may stress the value of routine trips to a primary care doctor or other healthcare professional. It could go over how primary care helps to manage general health, deal with issues, and offer the proper preventative care. It could also

emphasize how important it is to have a solid rapport with a healthcare professional.

3. Regular Health Screenings: The numerous health exams that are advised for women at various phases of life are covered in this section. Mammograms, Pap smears, bone density scans, blood pressure checks, cholesterol checks, diabetes checks, and STI checks are just a few examples of tests that may be included. It could describe the goal of every screening, the suggested timing, and any potential advantages of early detection.

4. Age-Specific Health Screenings: The chapter may discuss age-specific health screenings, addressing the changing healthcare needs of women at different phases of life. It could talk about things like blood sugar tests, cholesterol checks, colon cancer screening, cervical cancer screening, and breast cancer screening. Depending on a person's risk factors, family history, and personal health concerns, it could also cover additional pertinent exams.

5. Importance of Self-Examinations: The importance of self-examinations in preserving health is highlighted in this section. It could include advice on how to do self-breast exams, skin checks, and other self-evaluation procedures that enable women to actively maintain their health and look out for any changes or anomalies.

6. Health Promotion and Risk Reduction: The chapter may cover measures for health promotion and risk reduction, such as modifying one's lifestyle via stress reduction, regular exercise, good eating, and

quitting smoking. It could emphasize how these elements affect general health and wellbeing and offer helpful advice for implementing good habits into daily life.

7. Importance of Follow-up Care: This section stresses the need of maintaining screening and checkup appointments and heeding medical professionals' recommendations for additional testing or treatment. To address any detected health risks, it can go over the need of prompt interventions, continuing monitoring, and contact with healthcare experts.

This chapter attempts to encourage women to actively participate in their healthcare by emphasizing the value of routine checkups and health screenings. It offers details on age-appropriate tests, preventative care, and self-examinations to encourage early identification, lower health risks, and proactive health management. In order to preserve general health and identify any problems early, routine checkups and screenings are essential. This allows for prompt intervention and better health results.

# 7

# Aging with Grace

In Chapter 7, the topic of aging is discussed, and advice is given on how women should accept and deal with it in a graceful and upbeat way. It tackles the psychological, emotional, and social elements of aging while putting a strong emphasis on keeping a happy outlook, good lifestyle choices, and self-care. The following are some major subjects that this chapter may touch on:

Understanding the Aging Process: This section gives an overview of how the body and mind change as women age as well as the natural aging process. It could go through typical physical changes such skin aging, hormone changes, metabolic changes, and how aging affects bone health and cognitive function.

2. Maintaining Physical Health: The chapter may include techniques for doing so as women become older. It could go over the value of consistent exercise, wholesome eating, and weight control. Additionally, it could target certain aging-related health issues including controlling chronic illnesses, protecting cardiovascular health, and fostering flexibility and mobility.

3. Promoting Emotional Well-Being: In this part, we discuss how to promote emotional and mental health as we age. It could provide suggestions for handling stress, building resilience, and discovering meaning and fulfillment later in life. It could also deal with the emotional components of being older, such as handling change in life, grieving a loss, and keeping up positive connections.

4. Improving Cognitive Health: This section may go through techniques for preserving cognitive health and halting cognitive decline in older women. It could include practices like mental stimulation, lifelong learning, maintaining social connections, and establishing good lifestyle choices that support brain health.

5. Promoting good Relationships and Social ties: In this part, it is emphasized how crucial it is for older women to maintain good relationships and social ties. It could include suggestions for forging new connections, preserving old ones, and getting involved in social activities and support groups. The topic of loneliness, isolation, and the significance of social support in preserving general well-being may also be covered.

6. Embracing Body Image and Self-Acceptance: The chapter may touch on self-acceptance issues and body image issues in relation to aging. It could include suggestions for embracing physical change, developing self-confidence, and fostering a good body image. It may also address cultural pressures and aging-related prejudices and encourage women to appreciate themselves for reasons other than outward beauty.

7. Healthy Lifestyle Options: In this part, it is discussed how crucial it is for aging women to pursue healthy lifestyle options. It could go through things like eating a balanced diet, getting enough sleep, handling stress, abstaining from bad habits like smoking and binge drinking, and implementing self-care and relaxing methods into everyday life.

This chapter intends to educate women to approach aging with a positive mentality, prioritize self-care, and make decisions that support their physical, emotional, and social well-being by offering advice on aging gracefully. It stresses that becoming older is a normal part of life and gives doable methods for accepting aging with dignity, fortitude, and a sense of purpose.

**Aging well and longevity**

The topics of good aging and longevity are the main topics of chapter 8. It examines numerous aspects of general health and wellbeing as people age, emphasizing methods and lifestyle decisions that might foster vitality, independence, and a higher standard of living. The following are some major subjects that this chapter may touch on:

1. Understanding the Aging Process: This part gives a general overview of aging, including the physiological alterations that take place as people age. It could go through how aging is affected by genetics, way of life, and environmental factors. It also discusses the distinction between "biological age" and "chronological age," highlighting how aging is a dynamic and personal process.

2. good Lifestyle Habits: To encourage good aging, the chapter may place a strong emphasis on the value of forming healthy lifestyle habits. It could talk about things like eating a nutritious, well-balanced diet, exercising regularly, getting enough sleep, and successfully handling stress. The importance of healthy behaviors in avoiding chronic illnesses and sustaining cognitive function may also be covered.

3. Brain Health and Cognitive Fitness: In this part, we discuss how to keep our minds sharp as we age. It could include details on techniques and behaviors that promote brain health, such mental exercise, lifelong learning, social interaction, and brain stimulation. Additionally, it could go over the value of controlling long-term conditions that might impair cognitive function as well as the contribution a healthy lifestyle makes to maintaining cognitive ability.

4. Chronic Disease Prevention and Management: The chapter could cover methods for avoiding and controlling conditions including heart disease, diabetes, osteoporosis, and specific types of cancer that are frequently brought on by aging. The importance of routine health examinations, early illness identification, and disease management strategies, including adherence to medication and alterations in lifestyle, may be covered.

5. Social relationships and Community Engagement: The significance of social relationships and community involvement for good aging is emphasized in this section. It may go through the advantages of preserving friendships, taking part in social events, and being involved in a welcoming community. Additionally, it may address possible issues like loneliness and isolation and offer techniques for strengthening social relationships as people age.

6. Purposeful Aging and Lifelong Learning: This chapter may discuss the idea of purposeful aging as well as the value of continuing education and personal development in fostering an enriching and meaningful existence as people get older. It could go through the advantages of having hobbies, doing volunteer work, and making new resolutions and objectives.

7. Healthy Aging and Longevity Across Cultures: This section will explore various cultural perspectives on healthy aging and longevity. It will also look at customs and behaviors that support good health as people age. It could talk on the value of cultural sensitivity in

healthcare and how cross-cultural learning might improve practices for healthy aging.

This chapter intends to enable individuals to make educated decisions and adopt lifestyle behaviors that improve their well-being as they age by offering knowledge and advice on healthy aging and longevity. It encourages people to embrace the possibilities and challenges of aging with life and purpose by advocating a holistic perspective on aging that takes into account its physical, mental, and social facets.

## How to Maintain Cognitive Health

Emphasizes the significance of preserving cognitive health over the course of life and offers tips and techniques to encourage the best possible brain health and cognitive ability preservation. In addition to providing advice on lifestyle decisions and activities that boost cognitive well-being, it investigates many aspects that may have an influence on cognitive health. These are some important subjects that may be touched with in this chapter:

1. Understanding Cognitive Health: This part gives a general overview of cognitive health and the function of the brain in day-to-day activities. It describes the various facets of cognitive function, such as memory, attention, problem-solving, and linguistic abilities. Additionally, it may discriminate between possible cognitive problems and age-related decline in order to manage the typical cognitive changes that come with aging.

2. Nutrition for the Brain: The chapter may touch on how food affects our ability to think clearly. It examines how a healthy diet full of minerals, anti-oxidants, and omega-3 fatty acids affects how well the brain functions. It could emphasize particular foods, such berries, leafy greens, fatty fish, nuts, and seeds, that promote cognitive wellness.

3. Physical Activity and Cognitive Function: The relationship between physical activity and cognitive function is emphasized in this section. It examines the advantages of regular exercise for brain health, such as greater brain blood flow, higher neuroplasticity, and improved cognitive function. It could include suggestions on different types of exercise and their beneficial effects on cognitive health, including cardiovascular activities, strength training, and mind-body activities.

4. Mental Stimulation and Brain Exercises: To preserve cognitive health, the chapter may highlight the value of mental stimulation and performing brain exercises. It examines mental exercises including crossword puzzles, reading, picking up new abilities, and playing

musical instruments. It may also talk on the advantages of continuing education, participating in intriguing conversations, and seeking out novel experiences to keep the mind active.

5. Adequate Sleep and Cognitive Function: The importance of getting enough sleep is highlighted in this section. It investigates the link between poor sleep, cognitive deterioration, and memory issues. It might offer advice on how to improve sleep hygiene, create a regular sleep schedule, and deal with common sleep problems that could affect cognitive performance.

6. Purposeful Aging and Lifelong Learning: This chapter may discuss the idea of purposeful aging as well as the value of continuing education and personal development in fostering an enriching and meaningful existence as people get older. It could go through the advantages of having hobbies, doing volunteer work, and making new resolutions and objectives.

7. Healthy Aging and Longevity Across Cultures: This section will explore various cultural perspectives on healthy aging and longevity. It will also look at customs and behaviors that support good health as people age. It could talk on the value of cultural sensitivity in healthcare and how cross-cultural learning might improve practices for healthy aging.

8. Managing Chronic disorders and Cognitive Health: In this chapter, we may talk about how chronic disorders like diabetes, hypertension, and cardiovascular disease affect our cognitive

performance. It highlights how crucial it is to appropriately manage these illnesses in order to reduce the risk of cognitive deterioration. To promote physical and mental health, it could include advice on dietary changes, medication adherence, and routine checkups with the doctor.

This chapter intends to encourage people to take proactive measures in protecting their cognitive capacities and enhancing general brain function by offering advice on maintaining cognitive health. It highlights the need of adopting a comprehensive strategy that includes a balanced diet, regular physical activity, mental stimulation, rest, stress management, social interaction, and efficient management of chronic illnesses. By using these strategies, people can improve their cognitive health.

**The Sexual Health of Older Women**

For older women, sexual wellbeing is just as crucial to overall health as it is for younger ones. The sexual health and pleasure of women as they age must be addressed and prioritized, even if the subject may still be seen as somewhat taboo or ignored by society. Here are some important things to think about:

1. Physical Changes: As women become older, they go through a number of physical changes that might have an impact on their sexual health. For instance, menopause can cause vaginal dryness, vaginal wall weakening, and a reduction in natural lubrication. Uncomfortable alterations like this may occur during sexual activity.

It's critical to keep in mind that these changes are natural and that they may be controlled with the right actions.

2. Communication: It's important to have frank discussions with your spouse. Understanding may be cultivated and difficulties that may occur can be addressed by talking about wants, worries, and any physical or emotional changes. For problems to be solved and a satisfying sexual relationship to be maintained, both parties must be encouraging and understanding.

3. Medical Issues and Prescription Drugs: A variety of medical issues, including diabetes, cardiovascular disease, and hormone imbalances, can have an impact on sexual health. Antidepressants and blood pressure drugs, which are frequently used by older women, might also have adverse effects that affect sexual performance. It's crucial to speak with medical experts to comprehend these possible side effects and, if necessary, look into alternate solutions.

4. Pelvic Floor Health: It's crucial for sexual wellbeing to have healthy pelvic floors. Exercises for the pelvic floor, sometimes referred to as Kegel exercises, can assist to build up the muscles that support the organs in the pelvis and enhance sexual performance. Regularly performing these exercises can improve sexual arousal and lower the chance of incontinence.

5. Mental and Emotional Health: Sexual wellbeing is highly influenced by emotional and mental health. Women may encounter

changes in their body image, self-esteem, or intimacy issues as they become older. A better and more fulfilling sexual life can be facilitated by addressing these emotional components through counseling, therapy, or support groups.

6. Exploration and Pleasure: Older women ought to feel free to experiment with their bodies and their sexual inclinations. experimenting with self-indulgence methods, utilizing lubricants or sex toys, and experimenting with various sexual acts can support or improve sexual pleasure and satisfaction.

7. Routine Checkups: Regular trips to the doctor, particularly gynecologists, can assist address any particular issues or conditions pertaining to sexual wellbeing. These experts may offer advice, suggest suitable therapies, and address any queries or worries.

Keep in mind that maintaining sexual wellbeing is a private, personalized experience. One person's solution might not be suitable for another. As women get older, it's critical to place a high priority on open communication, self-care, and seeking expert advice when necessary.

*Management of Chronic Conditions and Lifestyle*

The phrase "chronic conditions" refers to persistent medical issues that need continuing care. Diabetes, heart disease, high blood pressure, asthma, rheumatoid arthritis, and chronic pain problems are a few examples that are frequently used. Effective management of chronic illnesses and enhancement of general wellbeing both depend on lifestyle management. Here are some important things to think about:

1. Healthy Eating: Managing chronic diseases requires a diet that is well-balanced. Consuming a range of nutrient-dense foods is crucial. These foods should include fruits, vegetables, whole grains, lean meats, and healthy fats. Working with a registered dietitian or other healthcare expert to create a custom meal plan that takes into account any dietary restrictions or other factors connected to the chronic disease may be useful.

2. Consistent Physical Activity: Regular physical activity has several advantages for treating chronic illnesses. It can help maintain a healthy weight, promote overall wellbeing, control blood sugar levels, and improve cardiovascular health. Before beginning an exercise program, it's crucial to pick physical activities that are appropriate for the person's talents and limits and to speak with a healthcare practitioner.

3. Medication Compliance: Maintaining compliance with prescribed drugs is essential for managing chronic diseases. It's crucial to take drugs as prescribed, adhere to the suggested dose schedule, and alert your doctor to any adverse effects or concerns. Adherence to drug regimens can be improved by using pill organizers or reminders.

4. Stress management: Because chronic illnesses can be physically and emotionally taxing, stress levels might rise. Deep breathing exercises, meditation, yoga, mindfulness, and participating in activities that encourage relaxation and stress reduction are all effective ways to manage stress. Emotional support can also be obtained by turning to family, friends, or support groups.

5. Getting Enough Sleep: Sleeping well is essential for general health and wellbeing. Chronic diseases can occasionally interfere with sleep habits, and inadequate sleep can exacerbate symptoms and make it harder to treat the condition. A regular sleep schedule, a cozy bedroom, and proper sleep hygiene are all things that can enhance the quality of your slumber.

5. Getting Enough Sleep: Sleeping well is essential for general health and wellbeing. Chronic diseases can occasionally interfere with sleep habits, and inadequate sleep can exacerbate symptoms and make it harder to treat the condition. A regular sleep schedule, a cozy bedroom, and proper sleep hygiene are all things that can enhance the quality of your slumber.

6. Avoiding Risky Behaviors: Some actions can aggravate long-term diseases or raise the possibility of complications. It's important to refrain from using tobacco products, consume alcohol in moderation in accordance with medical advice, and keep away from toxins or other chemicals that could exacerbate the disease.

7. Recurring Medical Exams: The course of a chronic ailment must be tracked regularly so that treatment strategies may be modified as necessary. Regular consultations with medical experts may help you spot any changes, get the right tests, and guarantee that the treatment plan is effective.

To create a thorough treatment plan that is suited to each patient's needs, it is crucial to collaborate closely with medical experts such primary care physicians, specialists, and allied health practitioners. Self-care and lifestyle modifications can considerably improve the management of chronic illnesses and improve overall quality of life when accompanied with the proper medical interventions.

# 8

# Society and Women's Health

The interplay between women's health and society has a significant influence on a variety of dimensions of women's well-being. Women's health is a crucial component of public health. In order to better understand how society and women's health interact, this chapter looks at the social, cultural, economic, and political aspects that affect women's health outcomes and experiences.

1. Gender Bias in Healthcare: Historically, gender biases have existed in the healthcare industry, and women's health issues have frequently been minimized or disregarded. This prejudice may lead to a delayed or ineffective diagnosis and course of therapy. There are initiatives underway to increase awareness of gender inequities in healthcare, advance gender-sensitive practices, and guarantee women's equal access to high-quality medical treatment.

2. Reproductive Health and Rights: Women's entire wellbeing is strongly influenced by their reproductive health. For women to exercise their reproductive rights and make educated decisions about their bodies and lives, they must have access to comprehensive reproductive healthcare services, such as family planning, contraception, prenatal care, safe abortion, and infertility therapies.

The availability and accessibility of these services are influenced by sociocultural variables and legislative choices.

3. Maternal Health: The well-being of women throughout pregnancy, delivery, and the postpartum period is the emphasis of maternal health. Maternal mortality and morbidity rates are influenced by socioeconomic variables, particularly in developing nations. These factors include poverty, poor access to healthcare, and a lack of education. Promoting prenatal care, having a qualified birth attendant present, providing emergency obstetric care, and addressing socioeconomic determinants of health are all actions taken to enhance mother health.

4. Violence Against Women: Female genital mutilation, sexual assault, and domestic abuse all have serious physical and psychological repercussions. These types of violence have their roots in society standards and gender inequity. Comprehensive methods incorporating legislative frameworks, awareness campaigns, support services, and initiatives to change cultural attitudes and behaviors are necessary to combat violence against women.

5. Mental health: Disorders of the mind include depression, anxiety, and eating disorders disproportionately impact women. These discrepancies are a result of a number of factors, including hormonal changes, reproductive experiences, gender-based violence, and social expectations. Destigmatizing mental illness, expanding access to mental health services, and including mental health into primary healthcare are all necessary for addressing women's mental health.

6. Health inequalities: Women from underrepresented and vulnerable groups, such as immigrants, LGBTQ+ people, racial and ethnic minorities, and women with disabilities, frequently encounter overlapping forms of discrimination and suffer from exacerbated health inequalities. Recognizing and correcting these inequities calls for an intersectional strategy that takes into account the particular difficulties that various groups of women confront.

7. Women's Empowerment and Health: Women's health outcomes are highly correlated with their level of empowerment, which includes their access to education, economic opportunity, and political engagement. Women who feel empowered are more likely to seek medical treatment, make educated health decisions, and fight for their rights. Improved health results are a result of initiatives to advance gender equality, do away with discriminatory behavior, and offer chances for women's empowerment.

8. Women's Health Policies and Advocacy: Addressing women's health challenges requires strong government policies and advocacy. Women's health outcomes are directly impacted by policies on

reproductive health, maternal health, violence prevention, gender equality, and healthcare finance. Women's health groups and activists engage in advocacy work to increase public awareness, influence legislation, and win funding for women's health programs.

The chapter emphasizes the intricate connection between society and women's health. The social determinants of health, gender biases, and structural injustices may be identified and addressed in order to improve the health of women, give women greater influence, and make society more egalitarian and inclusive. For long-lasting advances in women's health and wellbeing, cooperation between governments, healthcare providers, civil society groups, and people is essential.

**Rights of Women and Advocacy**

Women's rights advocacy entails work to advance and safeguard the equality, rights, and well-being of women in a variety of spheres of life. The social, political, economic, and legal sectors are included in this. The goal of women's rights activism is to confront and overcome gender-based violence, injustice, and discrimination. The following are important facets of women's rights and advocacy:

1. Legal Frameworks and Human Rights: Promoting women's rights frequently entails promoting the development, adoption, and enforcement of laws and regulations that safeguard women's human rights. Laws addressing, among other things, employment discrimination, gender equality in education, equal pay, and gender-

based violence are included in this. A foundation for protecting human rights is provided by international treaties like the Convention on the Elimination of All Forms of Discrimination Against Women (CEDAW). a foundation for advancing and defending women's rights internationally.

2. Combating gender-based violence, including as domestic abuse, sexual assault, female genital mutilation, and human trafficking, is a key issue of women's rights campaigning. Advocates attempt to change social attitudes that enable violence against women, reform judicial systems, and increase public awareness of the issue.

3. Reproductive Rights: The campaign for women's reproductive rights is focused on preserving women's autonomy and right to make decisions about their reproductive health. This include having access to safe abortion services, contraception, prenatal and postnatal care, prenatal and postnatal education, and complete sexual and reproductive healthcare. The goal of advocacy is to remove obstacles to reproductive rights, deal with stigma, and advance all-inclusive reproductive healthcare services.

4. Economic Empowerment: Promoting women's economic empowerment aims to remove economic discrimination against women and give them equal opportunity in the workforce. This entails speaking up in favor of laws that support parental leave, childcare that is affordable, equitable pay, and access to both formal and informal learning opportunities. It also discusses the obstacles

that women business owners confront and encourages the representation of women in positions of leadership.

5. Political involvement: Women's rights advocacy works to expand women's representation in politics and political involvement. This involves promoting election changes, helping women improve their leadership skills, and removing obstacles that prevent them from participating fully in public and political life. In governance and policy making, efforts are made to promote gender equality in representation and influence.

6. Intersectionality and Inclusivity: Advocates for women's rights acknowledge the overlapping forms of marginalization and discrimination experienced by women from a variety of backgrounds, including racial and ethnic minorities, LGBTQ+ people, indigenous women, women with disabilities, and migrant women. The goal of advocacy is to advance inclusive feminist movements by promoting intersectional strategies that meet the special needs and problems faced by all women.

7. Education and Awareness: Women's rights advocacy entails educating people about issues such as violence against women, discrimination against women, and gender inequity. It consists of educational campaigns, seminars, and community involvement to undermine gender stereotypes, advance gender equality, and equip people to speak out for women's rights in their neighborhoods. In order to raise awareness and mobilize support for women's rights, media involvement and internet platforms are also crucial.

8. Collaboration and Partnerships: Successful women's rights campaigning frequently entails cooperation between private citizens, governmental bodies, non-governmental groups, and international organizations. In order to advance women's rights and equality, partnerships with women's organizations, human rights organizations, grassroots movements, and governmental entities are strengthened. They also make it easier for people to work together in this endeavour.

Women's rights campaigning is a continuous and dynamic process that necessitates consistent efforts to remove institutional constraints and encourage radical change. Individuals and groups may help build a more just, inclusive, and equitable society by standing out for women's rights.


## Healthcare Access and Disparities

Healthcare disparities are inequalities in the availability of healthcare services, the standard of treatment, and the results of those services among various demographic groups. Numerous variables, including as socioeconomic position, race/ethnicity, gender, geography, age, and the presence of a handicap, might have an impact on these differences. Promoting health equality and enhancing general population health depend on addressing healthcare inequities and providing equitable access to healthcare. Here are some critical elements relating to access to care and healthcare disparities:

1. Socioeconomic Factors: Healthcare inequalities are significantly influenced by socioeconomic status. Due to financial limitations, a lack of health insurance coverage, and scarce resources, those with lower incomes, less education, or insecure work sometimes encounter difficulties to receiving healthcare. The implementation of safety net programs, the expansion of access to affordable health insurance, and the provision of financial aid for medical services are all actions taken to alleviate socioeconomic gaps in healthcare.

2. Disparities based on race and ethnicity: Access to and quality of healthcare is frequently uneven for people of color and ethnic minorities. These differences can be linked to a number of things, such as unconscious prejudice, discrimination, cultural and linguistic hurdles, and structural inequality. Culturally competent treatment, language access services, anti-discrimination laws, and initiatives to diversify the healthcare workforce are all necessary to address racial and ethnic inequities.

3. Geographical Inequalities: Access to healthcare might differ between urban and rural locations. A lack of healthcare professionals, a paucity of providers, and transportation issues are common problems for rural areas. The improvement of transportation choices for accessing healthcare as well as the expansion of telemedicine services are initiatives to overcome regional inequities.

4. Healthcare Disparities are influenced by gender, with women experiencing particular difficulties. Women's health requirements, such as maternity and reproductive care, might be disregarded or not sufficiently met. Additionally, the diagnosis, treatment, and research of some health disorders can be impacted by gender biases and preconceptions. In order to overcome gender inequities, it is critical to advance gender equity in healthcare, gender-sensitive healthcare services, and women's access to reproductive healthcare.

5. Health Literacy and Education: Healthcare disparities may be exacerbated by low health literacy, which is the capacity to comprehend and use health information and services. People with poor health literacy may find it difficult to obtain and use healthcare services efficiently, which has a negative impact on their health. This gap may be closed by improving health literacy through instruction, clear communication, and readily available health information.

6. Cultural Competence: Understanding and valuing the cultural customs, beliefs, and values of various people is necessary for cultural competence in healthcare. To give patients with the proper

treatment, healthcare organizations and systems must be aware of and receptive to their cultural demands. Cultural inequalities can be lessened by educating healthcare personnel about cultural competency, encouraging diversity in the healthcare sector, and implementing patient-centered methods.

7. Health System Reforms: The healthcare system has to be changed fundamentally in order to address healthcare inequities. This entails putting policies into place to increase access to healthcare, enhancing the safety net programs' funding, promoting health equity in research and clinical trials, and tracking and addressing disparities through data collection and analysis.

8. Community Engagement: It's important to include communities, especially underprivileged and marginalized ones, in order to comprehend their individual requirements, preferences, and barriers to healthcare access. Healthcare inequalities may be found and addressed locally by working with community groups, running outreach initiatives, and incorporating residents in decision-making processes.

It takes a multifaceted strategy combining governments, healthcare providers, communities, and individuals to lessen healthcare inequities and increase access. Progress may be achieved toward attaining health equality for all by addressing the underlying socioeconomic determinants of health, increasing equity in healthcare delivery, and making sure that everyone has the chance to obtain high-quality treatment.

## Safety and Gender-Based Violence

Any kind of violence that is primarily or solely directed at people based on their gender is referred to as gender-based violence. People of both genders are impacted by this profoundly ingrained social problem, but women and girls are disproportionately afflicted. Gender-based violence must be addressed, and safety must be ensured. This needs an all-encompassing strategy that incorporates people, communities, organizations, and governments. Key elements of gender-based violence and safety include the following:

1. Recognizing Gender-Based Violence: Gender-based violence takes many different forms, such as female genital mutilation, forced marriage, sexual assault, rape, intimate relationship abuse, harassment, and human trafficking. The fact that gender-based violence violates human rights and is a result of power disparities and gender inequality must be acknowledged.

2. Prevention and Education: Through education and awareness-raising campaigns, prevention efforts aim to address the underlying

causes of gender-based violence. Promoting gender equality and respect from an early age entails addressing negative gender conventions and stereotypes, encouraging healthy and respectful interactions, teaching consent, and encouraging bystander intervention.

3. Legal and Policy Frameworks: To combat gender-based violence, strong legal and policy frameworks must be established and enforced. All types of gender-based violence should be made illegal by law, and laws should also protect survivors and guarantee that offenders get just punishment. Prevention, survivor support services, reactions from the criminal system, and coordination amongst key parties should all be covered by comprehensive policies.

4. Support Services: For people impacted by gender-based violence, it's critical to offer accessible and survivor-focused support services. The establishment of hotlines, shelters, counseling services, medical assistance, legal assistance, and rehabilitation programs are all included in this. Support services should be customized to address the many needs of survivors, including those from underrepresented groups, LGBTQ+ people, and those with impairments.

5. Giving survivors the tools, support, and information they need to make their own decisions and reclaim control of their life is known as giving survivors the power. This includes access to economic possibilities, housing aid, help for education, and emotional and psychological support in addition to trauma-informed care.

Enhancing survivors' voices and including them in decision-making processes are further aspects of empowerment.

6. Modifying societal Norms: Confronting harmful societal attitudes and norms that support violence is essential to addressing gender-based violence. Promoting gender equality, respect, and consent in all spheres of society—including the classroom, the media, and popular culture—is part of this. Promoting healthy masculinity and avoiding violence requires including men and boys as friends and advocates.

7. Involving Communities: Preventing and treating gender-based violence depend heavily on community involvement. Communities are essential in establishing safe spaces, assisting survivors, and addressing harmful practices. Community leaders, groups, and grassroots movements working together can encourage group action and societal change.

8. worldwide Collaboration: Because gender-based violence is a worldwide problem, there must be global cooperation and collaboration. In order to exchange best practices, promote gender equality on international platforms, support programs addressing violence, and offer resources for preventative and response initiatives, governments, organizations, and civil society must collaborate.

In order to address gender-based violence and provide safety, a comprehensive strategy that addresses its core causes must be employed. We can work towards a society free from gender-based violence where everyone may live in safety and dignity through promoting gender equality, opposing damaging norms, helping survivors, and encouraging community involvement.

## Women's health and intersectionality

The term "intersectionality" describes how social constructs including gender, race, class, sexual orientation, disability, and other identities are intertwined. It acknowledges that people may encounter overlapping systems of prejudice and oppression as a result of their intersecting identities. Understanding how intersectionality affects health outcomes and experiences is crucial when looking at women's health. Key elements of intersectionality and women's health include the following:

1. Multiple kinds of Discrimination: Intersectionality shows how the overlapping kinds of discrimination experienced by women from marginalized groups provide special difficulties for them. Women of color, for instance, may experience socioeconomic inequality, racial discrimination, and gender-based discrimination that have an impact on their health outcomes. In order to address health inequalities, it is essential to comprehend these complex facets of discrimination.

2. Health gaps: Intersectionality has a role in the gaps in health that exist across various groups of women. Women who are members of disadvantaged groups, such as racial and ethnic minorities, LGBTQ+

people, people with disabilities, and immigrant women, frequently experience exacerbated health disparities. Social determinants of health, access to healthcare, discrimination within healthcare institutions, and cultural considerations can all have an impact on these differences.

3. Healthcare Access: Intersectionality affects who can access healthcare services. Language issues, cultural insensitivity, lack of health insurance, limited financial means, and prejudice in healthcare settings are just a few of the challenges that women from underprivileged backgrounds may encounter. These obstacles may make it more difficult for women to get the essential medical care, which might result in discrepancies in preventative care, early diagnosis, and prompt treatment.

4. Reproductive Health: Women's experiences and access to reproductive healthcare are significantly shaped by intersectionality. The availability of contraception, prenatal care, safe abortion services, fertility therapies, and information about reproductive health may differ for women from diverse ethnic and socioeconomic backgrounds. In order to better address the unique needs and obstacles experienced by various groups of women seeking reproductive healthcare, intersectional approaches are helpful.

5. Maternal Health: Intersectionality affects the results of maternal health. Preterm delivery, maternal death, and other unfavorable birth outcomes are frequently more common among women in marginalized groups, particularly women of color and those from

low-income families. Improving maternal health outcomes requires an understanding of the socioeconomic determinants of health, addressing racial and ethnic inequities, and offering treatment that is sensitive to cultural differences.

6. Mental Health: Women's mental health is impacted by intersectionality. Women from disadvantaged groups may be disproportionately affected by factors including racial discrimination, gender-based violence, financial inequality, and stigma. An intersectional strategy that takes into account the special needs and experiences of various women is necessary to address the inequities in mental health.

7. Empowerment and Advocacy: Intersectionality emphasizes the value of empowering women from underrepresented groups and amplifying their perspectives in discussions on healthcare. Health equity may be promoted, overlapping forms of discrimination can be addressed, and the unique issues encountered by different groups of women can be addressed through inclusive and representational advocacy initiatives.

8. Research and Data Collection: The importance of inclusive and thorough research on women's health is highlighted by intersectionality. Health inequalities may be found and addressed with the use of data collection that reflects overlapping identities and experiences. It enables a better knowledge of how diverse factors affect health outcomes and provides information for actions and policies that are supported by evidence.

An intersectional perspective on women's health recognizes the many needs and experiences of women from various backgrounds. Healthcare systems, policies, and advocacy initiatives may strive toward more equitable and inclusive healthcare services and improved health outcomes for all women by taking into account the overlapping elements that affect women's health.

**Giving future generations more authority**

Building a more inclusive, egalitarian, and sustainable society requires empowering future generations. It entails giving young people the information, know-how, tools, chances, and resources they need to realize their full potential and make valuable contributions to society. Key elements of enabling future generations are as follows:

1. Education: A vital component of empowerment is high-quality education. It gives young people the fundamental information, analytical abilities, and decision-making skills they need. Future generations must have access to inclusive and equitable education,

regardless of gender, financial position, or other identification markers.

2. Skill development: It's crucial to provide young people the skills they'll need for the future. Digital literacy, problem-solving, communication, teamwork, flexibility, and entrepreneurship are just a few examples of the academic and practical abilities that fall under this category. Young people can be empowered to navigate the changing labor market and seek fulfilling professions through skill development initiatives and vocational training programs.

3. Leadership Opportunities: Fostering leadership qualities and giving young people the chance to participate in decision-making processes are key components of empowering future generations. Student councils, youth parliaments, mentoring efforts, and youth-led programs can all help with this. Promoting youth involvement in community planning and policy-making strengthens their feeling of agency and gets them ready for future leadership positions.

4. Health and Well-Being: Encouraging young people's mental, emotional, and physical health is essential for their empowerment. The promotion of a healthy lifestyle, education on sexual and reproductive health, access to comprehensive healthcare services, and support for mental health are crucial elements. Giving young people the knowledge and tools to make smart health decisions benefits their general success and well-being.

5. Financial Literacy and Economic Empowerment: Giving young people the knowledge and tools necessary for financial literacy while also fostering economic possibilities gives them the ability to become financially independent and make wise financial decisions. This involves offering access to entrepreneurial programs, coaching, and internships, as well as teaching budgeting, saving, and investment skills.

6. Social Justice and Civic Engagement: Encouraging youth to actively participate in civic affairs and promote social justice causes equips them to be change agents. Their feeling of social responsibility is strengthened and they are given the tools they need to take on society difficulties when the ideals of equality, inclusiveness, human rights, and environmental sustainability are promoted.

7. Mentorship and Role Models: Young people's personal and professional growth may be greatly impacted by mentoring programs that pair them with seasoned professionals and good role models. Mentors offer advice, encouragement, and inspiration to young people, assisting them in overcoming obstacles, establishing objectives, and developing resilience.

8. Promoting invention and Creativity: Promoting a culture of invention, creativity, and entrepreneurship is essential to empowering future generations. Young people may better the future by being encouraged to think critically, take calculated risks, and

come up with creative solutions to social, environmental, and economic problems.

9. Environmental Awareness: In order to empower future generations, it is essential to teach children about environmental sustainability and to promote Eco-friendly actions. Instilling a feeling of responsibility for the earth and empowering young people to participate in the creation of a more sustainable future are two benefits of promoting sustainable habits, climate action, and environmental stewardship.

10. Dismantling Gender preconceptions: Dismantling gender preconceptions is essential to empowering future generations. Young people may better understand their rights, confront prejudice, and advance a more fair society by supporting gender equality, inclusion, and respect for all genders.

Governments, educational institutions, families, communities, and numerous stakeholders all work together in a continual endeavor to empower future generations. We can build a better future where everyone has the chance to prosper and make a significant contribution to society by investing in the empowerment of young people.

# 9

# Conclusion

For women's general wellbeing as well as the wellbeing of society as a whole, it is essential to provide them the tools they need to take control of their health. Giving women the information, tools, and support they need to make educated decisions about their health and to speak out for their needs is a crucial part of empowering them in the healthcare industry. We can advance gender equality, enhance health outcomes, and build a more inclusive and fair healthcare system by empowering women in the field of medicine.

Focusing on a few key areas is crucial if we want to empower women in the healthcare industry. First and foremost, it is crucial to encourage access to comprehensive and reasonably priced healthcare services. Access to preventative care, treatment for physical and mental health disorders, maternity healthcare, and reproductive healthcare are all included in this. To provide equal access for all women, it also entails addressing healthcare inequities, such as those based on race, socioeconomic position, and region.

Second, it is crucial to spread knowledge and information concerning women's health. Women should have access to precise, factual information on their bodies, reproductive health, menstrual health, menopause, and other particular health issues. Women who have access to education are more equipped to make wise health decisions, find the right treatment, and take an active role in their healthcare.

Third, it is critical to encourage women to participate in healthcare decision-making. Women should be given the chance to take part in talks about their treatment options, take part in research studies, and have their opinions heard in the procedures that determine policy. In order to create healthcare policies and services that best serve women's particular needs, women's ideas and experiences are crucial.

It's also critical to overcome gender biases and prejudices in healthcare systems. Training in gender-sensitive care, cultural sensitivity, and knowledge of the various needs and experiences of women should be provided to healthcare professionals. This may make sure that women receive treatment that is appropriate for their needs and that they are treated with respect, decency, and understanding.

Moreover, it is crucial to develop surroundings that are supportive to women's health. The promotion of work-life balance, adaptable work schedules, and laws supporting women's reproductive health, such those allowing for parental leave and lactation accommodations, are a few examples of this. Addressing gender-based violence, offering assistance to survivors, and promoting a culture of safety and respect are all components of supportive settings.

In the end, encouraging women to take control of their health is a complex task that calls for cooperation between people, healthcare professionals, decision-makers, and communities. We can improve the lives of women and contribute to a more just and healthy society by empowering them in the healthcare industry. Women who are empowered may make wise decisions, stand up for their rights, and live longer, happier lives.